DEFYING
THE GODS

■

Also by Scott McCartney

Trinity's Children: Living Along America's Nuclear
Highway (with Tad Bartimus)

DEFYING
THE GODS

INSIDE THE NEW FRONTIERS
OF ORGAN TRANSPLANTS

SCOTT MCCARTNEY

A LISA DREW BOOK
Macmillan Publishing Company
New York

Maxwell Macmillan Canada
Toronto

Maxwell Macmillan International
New York   Oxford   Singapore   Sydney

Lisa Drew Books
Macmillan Publishing Company
866 Third Avenue
New York, NY 10022

Maxwell Macmillan Canada, Inc.
1200 Eglinton Avenue East
Suite 200
Don Mills, Ontario M3C 3N1

Macmillan Publishing Company is part of the Maxwell Communication Group of Companies.

"Mercy Mercy Me (The Ecology)" by Marvin Gaye, © 1971, Jobete Music Co., Inc. Reprinted by permission.

Library of Congress Cataloging-in-Publication Data
McCartney, Scott.
Defying the gods: inside the new frontiers of organ transplants/Scott McCartney.
p.   cm.
"A Lisa Drew Book."
Includes bibliographical references.
ISBN 0-02-582820-7
1. Liver—Transplantation—Popular works.   2. Liver—Transplantation—Case studies.   I. Title.
RD546.M34   1994
617.5'56—dc20   93-38976
CIP

Macmillan books are available at special discounts for bulk purchases for sales promotions, premiums, fund-raising, or educational use. For details, contact:

Special Sales Director
Macmillan Publishing Company
866 Third Avenue
New York, NY 10022

10 9 8 7 6 5 4 3 2 1

Printed in the United States of America

■

In Pam's memory

CONTENTS

ACKNOWLEDGMENTS

This book never would have been possible without the trust and courage of the doctors and patients profiled here. They have my utmost admiration for their compassion, their skill, their convictions. Most of all, they believed the project would be beneficial toward promoting good public policy and greater understanding about organ donation.

Goran Klintmalm never hesitated to allow me inside his world and opened the door wide. No author has ever had a more gracious, more professional host. In the operating room, in the office, in the hallways, he and his team could not have been more accommodating or caring about the project. Robert Goldstein was supportive from the start. Marlon Levy was an instant friend, thoughtful, open, funny, and wise. Bo Husberg couldn't have been more amenable on several all-night donor runs.

My desk and my allegiances at Transplant Services quickly fell in line with the four fellows: Dale Distant, Caren Eisenstein, Tom Renard, and senior fellow Lars Backman. All are terrific surgeons and wonderful doctors with bright futures ahead. The third generation of transplantation—or whatever field they land in—will be in good hands.

I came to rely heavily on the transplant program's four coordinators, each a high-octane mixture of insightful nurse, wise counselor, and master drill sergeant. I shared special bonds with some who had cared for my sister-in-law during her ordeal. I owe many thanks to Sharon Anderson, Sharon Carlen, Pam Fertig, and Donna Morrissey.

Alison Victoria, who lives a schizophrenic life of dexterous hospital bureaucrat and imaginative artist, earns deep respect from patients for her skill and advocacy at negotiating the financial and insurance maze. I am no different. She was a terrific confidante and helpful angel, and her care and warmth shone through the photographs she took for this book.

I received tremendous support and cooperation from social workers, nurses, researchers, chaplains, dietitians, and secretaries at Baylor, especially Michelle Long, Leslie Stoneman, Karen Smith, Grady Hinton, Chris Morris, Tom Haycraft, Jean Balthazor, Isaac Watemberg, Tina Dawald, Jeanette Hasse, Linda Blue, Kathy O'Dea, Janel McDonald, Ruth Black, Vy Malcik, Judy Price, and Shaylor Adams. Dr. Daniel Polter allowed me into the selection committee with the same respect and openness he delivers to all his patients. I was allowed to attend four months of meetings on the grounds only that I protect the specific identity of most opinions—in most cases, no names attached to what was said. Dr. Polter provided prescient wisdom along the way, as did Doctors Tom Gonwa, Martin Mai, Jeff Crippin, Dan DeMarco, Harry Sarles, and Mike Ramsay. John Wallace, Cindy Morphew, Allison Smith, and the folks at the Southwest Organ Bank in Dallas were of great help.

Tom Starzl was a delight to get to know and a challenging and invigorating source through the exhilaration of his baboon transplant days as well as the rigors of controversy over the speedy transplantation of the governor of Pennsylvania. His dedication and brilliance is an inspiration, his pioneering work has saved many, many lives, and his own book, *The Puzzle People: Memories of a Transplant Surgeon*, is a remarkable achievement as well. If the test for us all is whether we made a difference, then Tom Starzl stands very tall: He has made a titanic difference.

Friends, colleagues, and family offered advice and tips. Hal Lancaster and Paul Steiger of the *Wall Street Journal* adopted me and this book with grace. Carol Mann recognized the project right away and, once again, helped me focus my idea into something workable. Lisa Drew picked it up with great enthusiasm and potent support. She turned me loose then saved me from my clichés. Her assistant, Katherine Boyle, was also a solid, careful editor and great help. My father, Alan, a gastroenterologist who always spiced the dinner table talk with tales of liver biopsies and ulcers, was a valuable sounding board. Once again, Tad Bartimus helped keep me on course, reading early drafts and pushing me as always to do better, while offering the kind of crucial nourishment only best friends can deliver.

As always, my wife, Karen Blumenthal, was tremendously supportive and sterling in her editorial help, even if she did get chocolate all over the manuscript. Pat Ashworth kept us all together, and Bob and Beverly Blumenthal were always there. For the family, this was the most painful project I could have ever attempted. No one discouraged; everyone always believed.

Most of all, though, my gratitude goes to the people who adopted me into their families at a time of unbelievable crisis. The patients profiled in this book all unselfishly shared themselves so that others might learn. Don and Cathy Bryan, Cynthy and Randy Roady, Connie and Mel Berg, and Arden Lynn, her son Robert and daughter Sue, all found the strength to trust in me and believe in the book.

This book is dedicated to the memory of Dr. Pam Blumenthal, who helped many souls in her too-short life. We miss her very much. But it is really a tribute to all, including Pam, who try to defy the gods.

INTRODUCTION

The stories are heard so often that they seem almost commonplace, part of our standard medical diet. The top executive at MCI disappears for a few weeks and returns with a new heart. A new liver saves the life of a young mother; a child with cystic fibrosis waits for new lungs; a diabetic waits for a new pancreas; a hepatitis victim gets a liver from a baboon; the governor of Pennsylvania receives a new heart and liver. Stormie Jones grows from a child to a teenager with someone else's heart and liver. Tiny Charlie Fourstar puts on ballet slippers and pirouettes with five new organs inside her, a completely transplanted belly.

It seems so simple: Got a dying organ? Get a new one.

It's not, of course. Replacing human organs like some auto mechanic dropping in a new carburetor is one of the most spectacular of all human endeavors. It's still among the most challenging fields of modern medicine, attracting the best and most daring of the healers, who offer cures for incurable diseases. Their world is one where normal rules don't apply or haven't been made up yet. The reality is that they remake human bodies, over and over again. And the emotions are always near the surface: Triumph is the inducement, but tragedy is a necessary part of the process.

■

For while transplantation offers hope for people who have used up all their chances with God, it also presents terrible choices for families and ethical dilemmas for physicians. Someone must die so that someone may live. Choices must be made, for there are far fewer donor organs than dying people. And while talented surgeons have mastered the art of replacing crucial organs, they haven't tamed the human body's natural instinct to reject them.

Beneath the headlines spin endless stories of courage and frustration, conquest and defeat. Our society's most highly skilled surgeons and their sickest patients carry on an intricate dance with death, hoping to defy the gods long enough to grant people a little more time with their friends, a few more birthday celebrations.

The process, and thus this book, is a medical adventure story, one with plenty of invisible killers and real-life heroes and villains, unlikely rescuers and terrible tragedies. Like most adventure stories, it is a tale of people stretching limits and even breaking laws—the laws of nature—to do the right thing.

For four months I became part of the liver and kidney transplant team at Baylor University Medical Center in Dallas, one of the biggest and best programs in the country. I was given complete and perhaps unprecedented access to everything that went on. I rode with teams of daredevil doctors on all-night plane rides to retrieve organs. I watched in the operating room through hours of surgery. I made rounds every day, attended meetings every week, sat in the pathology lab and examined biopsy slides, tagged along with chaplains and social workers, even took a drug salesman or two for a free lunch. I became friend, researcher, chronicler.

I also sat with families for hours of praying and waiting and hoping, becoming part of their extended circle, sharing their victories and setbacks. I joined the patient's support group, hung out in the intensive care waiting room, impatiently waited for the day's lab report when it was delivered to the patient's room. Four different people, ranging in age from thirty-eight to sixty-eight, agreed to let me go through the ordeal of receiving a liver transplant with them, sharing all dimensions of this most profound experience—the emotional, the medical, the mechanical, the unexplainable. As they did, I wore a beeper nervously awaiting the call that a liver had been found for them and even found myself secretly, morbidly, hoping that a holiday weekend might produce a donor.

This book was written as the events occurred, without knowing who would live and who would die. It was completed a year after the patients' transplants. Most of the existing reportage and literature on transplants has focused on the dramatic surgery and ended there. But that is only the beginning. The hardest part is no longer simply sewing in a new liver. It is finding a way to convince the body that the liver should be accepted and convincing the new liver that it should work properly, balancing bodily functions for a new host with different needs. The surgery is not the hardest part; the recovery is.

Intertwined are some of the most pressing public policy issues of the day. Transplants are one reason why health-care costs are skyrocketing; what will the nation do about that? Will the day come when we can no longer afford the best treatments and the most exciting research? For many, lacking insurance or government assistance, that day is already here. Hundreds are turned away from transplant centers simply because they can't afford the $200,000 price tag. And some patients die waiting for a transplant, even when healthy organs are available. On the same day that someone near death in an intensive care unit is supposedly listed in a nationwide computer data bank as first-priority, emergency priority, another relatively healthy patient of the same size and blood type might get a liver that would be perfect for either. Why? Where does the system break down, and what can be done to fix it?

This was not the first time I had been through the transplant experience. Three years earlier, my sister-in-law

Pam received a liver, kidney, and pancreas from the same Baylor team. She was the first patient to receive those three organs, and as it is for all transplant patients, it was her only hope. She had almost died when she was in graduate school, and had courageously lived the next decade chronically ill, knowing that someday a transplant would be her only hope for a normal life. Everything began terrifically after the surgery, which occurred five years to the day after Baylor dramatically launched its program by handling an emergency transplant for a five-year-old girl who had captured national headlines and Nancy Reagan's attention. But after a few weeks post-transplant, Pam was inexplicably sick. By the time a fungal infection was discovered, it was too late to reverse its course.

Even being "twice blessed" was not enough. "I need more chances. More chances," she cried as she slipped into a coma. She died at age thirty-four, seven weeks to the day after her transplant.

Those ups and downs, our giddiness and tears, convinced me that there were incredible tales of survival and sacrifice to be told in this unseen world of transplantation. What I learned from Pam, and from the people kind enough to let me enter their lives, is how hard people will fight to stay alive and how hard others will fight to give them a second chance. In short, their stories are stories of the strength of the human spirit, the hunger to live and the value of life.

AUTHOR'S NOTE

To protect the privacy of families and patients, a few of the last names in this book have been changed as requested. All last names of organ donors have also been changed in keeping with privacy policies of organ banks and surgeons, who inform organ recipients only of their donors' age, sex, location, and cause of death.

■

DEFYING

THE GODS

CHAPTER 1
THE CHOICE

The phone rang early, catching Arden Lynn in the bathroom halfway between the dreams of sleep and the reality of morning. She dreaded this day, on which she had to close the financial books on the estates of her father, who died just before last Christmas, and of her husband, who died just nine days later in bed beside her. Somehow, on this warm Texas October morning, being a bit pokey in the bathroom seemed the safest thing to do.

Closing both estates was a race against the clock, for Lynn, too, was dying. She had been sick since 1980, progressively losing her energy as her skin turned more and more yellow. Her doctor told her that her liver was failing because the ducts that carry bile within it were collapsing, and the organ was choking itself to death. She was tired all the time, and fluid was building in her belly. Only fifty-nine years old in 1992, she was frightened she would no longer be able to live alone and take care of herself.

Like many other liver diseases, there was no cure for this, only treatment to postpone the inevitable. The liver—the body's chemical manufacturing plant—can control everything from food digestion to brain functioning, about five hundred functions in all. It is the carburetor of the engine. It provides energy sources to the rest of the body, makes protein and albumin, and gets rid of impurities. It is essential, and yet the

1

human body, blessed with two lungs, two eyes, two ears, even two kidneys, has only one liver. And while science has produced artificial hearts and artificial kidneys, manufacturing a liver—even "liver dialysis"—has remained an elusive and unsolvable puzzle. About half a million Americans suffer from liver disease, and each year, 35,000 die from it—almost as many as are killed on highways now. It is the nation's fourth worst killer disease, behind heart disease, strokes, and cancer.

Arden Lynn's only hope was getting a new liver, one from someone else.

In the intensive care unit (ICU) at Baylor University Medical Center in Dallas, a forty-six-year-old Hispanic grandmother lay in a coma, stricken by massive hepatitis that in just a couple of weeks had killed her liver. It was a lightning bolt, a virus so powerful, so much more potent than even the AIDS virus, that it can conk an otherwise healthy person out in just a few days. No one knew where the hepatitis A, the kind common in food poisoning, had come from. Doctors thought her highest risk came from her grandson, who was in day care, but that was a slim theory at best. Four weeks before, Yolanda Contreras had been perfectly healthy, a fun-loving five-feet-five, 130-pound school secretary who knew everyone in the neighborhood, everyone in her church. She and her husband had just celebrated their wedding anniversary. Now her eyes were like those of a doll; she had fever possibly related to pneumonia. Seizures were continuing. Doctors said she was within hours of death.

A debate was raging at Yolanda Contreras's bedside. Some doctors thought she was too far gone to attempt a liver transplant—a *tour de force* of modern surgery that takes anywhere from five to twenty hours. She had been airlifted to Baylor five days earlier on a three-hour helicopter flight from San Antonio, where she loved to volunteer with the PTA and school band programs. San Antonio had recently started a liver transplant program, but Contreras's condition was so serious, doctors suggested the transfer to Baylor. As she left, doctors told her husband she had a fifty-fifty chance of survival. "I was stunned, going from a little bout of hepatitis to almost dead in a matter of days," recalled her husband, John Contreras.

Ten years ago, there would have been no hope for either Arden Lynn or Yolanda Contreras. Just ten years ago, liver transplanting was in its infancy, barely accepted by the medical establishment, still unable to justify its benefit to those who finance health care. Now, however, there was at least hope. Transplanting organs allowed dying people to exchange one condition for another, relieving whatever disease was life-threatening, but introducing new dangers—from damage to other organs to increased risk of cancer, infections, and viruses. Overall, transplants improved quality of life and usually added some years to that life. New drugs made it possible. New techniques made it probable. It didn't always work, but the impossible was seductively becoming the routine. Now hospitals around the country were scurrying to establish transplant centers. Now the surgeons who perform these medical miracles had become the new purveyors of hope, offering cures to the dying, a second chance to those who had seemingly used up all their chances.

If nothing else, now there was hope.

Yolanda Contreras had arrived at Baylor barely conscious and soon slipped into a coma. Debate began immediately over whether even to put her on the nationwide emergency list for a liver. Fluid had accumulated in her skull, raising the pressure and making it harder and harder for her heart to pump blood into the brain. Without blood, the brain dies. Tests indicated that blood flow to the brain was diminished—but there was still flow. There was still a possibility she might not yet be brain damaged and, with a new liver, might recover fully.

On the other hand, if she was too unstable to survive the

surgery, a healthy liver might be lost. Survival of the liver, as well as the patient, must be considered because of the organ shortage, now at crisis proportions. Organ donations have been dropping in the United States for the past five years, partly because of better laws on seat belts and motorcycle helmets, partly because of air bags and other improved safety features in automobiles, and partly because emergency rooms rarely see single gunshot wounds to the head. Shooting victims these days come in sprayed with bullets from automatic weapons. And as liver transplanting has gained more acceptance, and become more lucrative, more and more hospitals across the country have established their own programs, scarfing up local livers in the process that otherwise might be flown off to far sicker patients at major transplant programs such as Baylor, Pittsburgh, and UCLA. The nation's system of organ banks offers livers first to local programs, regardless of the dying-patient priority. Then, if there are no local takers, the donated organ is offered for placement through the nationwide computer.

At Baylor, the second-largest adult liver transplant center in the country, with the highest survival rate of all major programs, more than fifty people routinely are on the waiting list. The wait used to be two weeks but now stretches up to and beyond four and five months. A few die waiting, a disturbingly more frequent occurrence. A healthy liver must not be wasted.

There were additional considerations. What if Yolanda Contreras did survive and turned out to be brain damaged? Was the surgeon doing her and her family any heroic favors?

The Baylor team explained their dilemma to the large and loving Contreras family gathered in the waiting room, a dark, open space with pink walls that had become a sanctuary of sorrow, or hope, for families enduring round-the-clock vigils.

"They never built up false hope. For that I am grateful," John Contreras said later. The buttoned-down, tall, handsome entrepreneur, his black hair accented by gray on the temples, runs his own beauty-products distribution company. Now he was eating and sleeping in the ICU waiting room, hanging on every word from the doctors, listening intently with his arms crossed, never outwardly losing control.

"I talked with the kids. We were already deciding what she would wear when we buried her and what to do with her rings," he said.

The family stared at the team of doctors with mournful, frightened faces. She could be dead before nightfall, they told Yolanda's family.

"I'll take her any way I can get her back," John Contreras replied. "Please, do something. . . . Please do something. . . ."

"She may not be the same Yolanda. . . ."

"I know. I'll take her any way I can get her back. Do the best you can."

The decision was made to list Yolanda in the national organ bank computer, a "status four," meaning she was in intensive care, needing life-support equipment to breathe, and likely to die within a matter of hours. Baylor would take a liver from any blood-type donor. Transplant surgeons usually match blood groups between recipient and donor, but in a case like this, the Baylor team decided to try anything.

A day went by with no calls about an organ, with Yolanda Contreras still clinging to life. Then another. Then another. At a regular meeting on Wednesday, seventy-two hours after she had been listed, the transplant team was aghast at the lack of livers. "I know everyone's aware of this, but I just wanted to say this is really frightening," said Jeff Crippin, a liver specialist.

That night, Baylor got a call. A fourteen-year-old donor was available in San Antonio, and the liver happened to be the right size and blood type, O, for Yolanda Contreras. Actually two donors were available that night, and the "harvest" team made an all-night journey around Texas.

With the liver in hand waiting in the operating room in an ice-filled Coleman cooler, the transplant team again began to decide if Yolanda Contreras could pass muster. Some wanted to do a special brain-pressure test where a bolt is screwed into the skull to measure pressure. But Baylor's neurosurgeons refuse to do that test in liver-failure patients because their blood has trouble clotting—clotting factors come from the liver—and the patient might bleed to death inside the brain.

The wall-mounted television above her bedside flickered twenty-four hours a day, even though the woman lying below was oblivious, closer to death than to life. The television is not for the patient, but for the doctors and nurses working in the ICU. TV noise is something to break the friction created by environment, a cacophony of beeps and buzzes from monitors, pumps, and ventilators. In the operating room, during the tension and pressure of transplant surgery, music becomes an anesthetic for the surgeons, who cut and sew to a range of tastes from rock to classical to Christian. But in the ICU, there is only the television, and without its sound, the beeps and buzzes become sonic torture, an audible slow drip of water on the face. As the discussion boiled at Yolanda Contreras's bedside, the game show "Jeopardy" was on. At piercing and poignant moments in the ICU, it can seem like "Jeopardy" is always on. Its theme song had imperceptibly become part of the routine. "Do do, do do, do do doo. . . ."

Dr. Goran Klintmalm, the head of Baylor's transplant program, who just a day earlier had told other doctors he didn't think Contreras should be on the list for a liver, ordered more tests, trying to be as methodical and scientific as possible. Over the summer, he had put a new liver in a young hepatitis patient in a coma, and she had awakened and was doing fine. But just the week before, a comatose older woman flown to Baylor from Oklahoma had not awakened after her transplant and appeared to be living only because of the ventilator that breathed for her. She was a constant reminder, just two doors down in the same ICU ward.

Test after test on Yolanda Contreras came up inconclusive. There would be no easy answer.

Since 1984, when he launched Baylor's transplant program with the father of liver transplants, Dr. Thomas Starzl, Klintmalm has had to make God-like decisions dozens and dozens of times. Not so much "playing God" as "practicing God," Klintmalm many times has chosen who will live, and who will die. Along with the glory of saving lives comes the pain of ending them. He, like all other transplant surgeons, finds ways to cope with the pain of the profession and ways to rationalize its failures and successes.

"It's always difficult to condemn a patient to death. It's a very tough decision to make," Klintmalm would recall later. "It's a difficult role, but we have to do it. If it's [the transplant] not going to work, then it's cruel to the patient, cruel to the family, and a waste of a liver. These decisions get tougher as livers get scarcer, and she was a very tough decision. She had a large family there. It's very difficult to say, 'No, you're not going to try,' when there's no absolute sign it won't work."

"Hello," Arden Lynn said, stumbling from the bathroom.

"Mrs. Lynn? This is Donna from Transplant Services at Baylor. How long will it take you to get to the hospital?"

Lynn was stunned. She had been told in the spring that she needed a new liver, but had dragged her feet. The stress of losing first her father, then her husband, of being told she, too, was dying, was overwhelming. On top of that, her son had been laid off last winter, her son-in-law had lost his job in June, her daughter had lost hers in August. It was all too much to deal with at once, but her illness kept reminding her that she had better get it done. Finally, convinced she needed the transplant, she got on the waiting list and carried a beeper for three months—so long that she had first convinced herself she would never get the call that a liver had been found for her. But in the last two or three days, something intangible had changed and she had begun believing that her time was coming. She had fingered her beeper more carefully lately, been a bit more nervous about it—even taking it in the bathroom when she showered. Just in case. She had begun to believe that the day would come soon, mostly because she was close to burying her past—something she had to do before turning to her future. She just needed one more day to close the books.

Her thoughts began racing as she listened in her half-awake, fuzzy state to Donna Morrissey, one of the coordinators for Klintmalm's program who helps keep the wheels rolling, beeping new patients, scheduling operating rooms, ordering medication, tracking old patients, teaching new ones how to care for their new bodies.

"I have to go to my accountant today," Arden thought to herself. "This is the last day. . . . I'm almost ready for this . . . I just need one more day to get ready. . . ."

Arden's hands were shaking.

"Forty minutes, I guess," she told Donna.

"No," Morrissey replied firmly. "Get in the car NOW."

"I have to call my daughter—"

"GET IN THE CAR NOW!"

The surgeons' decision had been to play "liver roulette." Yolanda Contreras would get a chance, but they were convinced that she would not survive the surgery and in fact might die even before the operation began. Klintmalm had told Pam Fertig, another of Baylor's transplant coordinators, that he was willing to go as far as putting the liver in Contreras, hooking it up and trying to start blood flow through it—the most crucial step for the patient. Unstable, a patient such as Contreras would surely not make it through the change in pressure that comes from uncrimping all the garden hoses of blood inside the

■

body. If she crashed, then Klintmalm would "reharvest" the liver and use it for the patient called in as "backup."

"That's never been done before," Kathryn O'Dea, one of the transplant team nurses, remarked. "But with these guys, that doesn't mean they won't try." So convinced was he that Contreras might die at any moment that Klintmalm told Morrissey he wanted the backup who could get to Baylor the quickest.

They looked down the waiting list, the "bible" of the transplant unit. On call and off, each coordinator and each surgeon carries the waiting list at all times.

"Arden Lynn is in Dallas."

"Don Bryan is sicker. He's from West Texas but is staying with relatives in Dallas."

Bryan, a rancher who had risen through the ranks of American Petrofina oil company only to clash with a new president and find early retirement, had been hospitalized for a couple of weeks with a belly full of ascites—fluid that accumulates because the liver is failing. Bedridden and weak, Bryan looked like a pregnant grandfather. At sixty-two, he could be taken for eighty-two. He had lost fifty pounds and now was skinny as an expectant fencepost at six-feet-two and only 124 pounds. Anxious for a liver, cranky from the illness, Bryan was a picture of misery. His wife and family were hanging on every phone call, scared that Don would die before a liver was found for him.

"Arden is closer, I think," Morrissey said.

"Call in Arden Lynn," Klintmalm ordered.

Actually, Arden Lynn and Don Bryan, who had gone through the evaluation process to get on the waiting list together and had become fast friends, were living within a few blocks of each other in the same Lake Highlands neighborhood of Dallas. She was listed first on the waiting list because her financial clearance—you have to prove you can pay before you're listed—had come four days quicker.

"We thought she was closer," Morrissey said later. "Then she said it would take forty minutes. Sometimes you have to be really firm with the patients. It's understandable. They get scared and start to stall."

On the fourteenth floor of the elegant seventeen-story hospital building, a floor of thirty-four beds devoted to liver and kidney transplant patients that is almost always full, Lynn learned the details of the life-and-death drama in which she had just been cast in a starring role.

Klintmalm, wearing clogs and green surgical scrubs, his wedding rings and Swedish Army dog tag hanging from a gold neck chain, shook hands and explained the situation. He had been up most of the night, a night that actually proved to be the start of a six-day marathon crush of round-the-clock work—seven livers and two kidneys over the next six days. Klintmalm first flew to San Antonio to harvest one liver and ship it back to Dallas in a second jet, then flew on to Austin to harvest a second liver of a different blood type. Then, after a catnap, he awoke to The Decision. Despite the fatigue, "GK," as he is known around the hospital, still looked like he had just come off the cover of "GQ."

"There is a woman who is very sick, in a coma, and we don't really think she can tolerate the surgery," Klintmalm told Lynn. "But we are going to start, going to give her every chance, and see how she does. If she does not do well, we will prep you for surgery and you will get the liver. So just wait, we should know something one way or another within an hour or two . . ."

"Do a good job," Arden said to Klintmalm as he wheeled around toward the elevators, stopping long enough to shoot back a quizzical glance at his patient.

"I don't think he thought that was too funny," Lynn said, rifling out her words while "high" on a potent combina-

■

tion of adrenaline and fear. "He's so young. He's so young. That was God, wasn't it?"

Arden Lynn was a gumbo of emotion. She immediately began worrying about the mother who had to die if she were to get her chance that day. "How many kids does she have? . . . How old is she? . . . Where's she from? . . . I really feel for that other family. . . ." She began thinking about the donor of the liver, the teenager in San Antonio who died the day before and whose family had the kindness to donate organs to help others. "It has bothered me all through this that somebody else has to die for me," Lynn said.

And she began worrying about Don Bryan, who she knew was having real problems. "He needs it worse than I do. He's so much sicker. I wonder why they called me and not him? I so wanted Don to go first."

Then she began worrying about her own possible surgery, something she was praying for but still dreading. Five years previously doctors routed some blood flow away from her liver by hooking up an emergency "shunt" in order to take some strain off the organ and keep it going awhile longer. The operation had lasted eight hours and "everybody in my family just about lost it. It didn't help much that the lady across the hall went down for the same surgery and didn't come back up," she said.

A transplant was considered at the time—1987—but the procedure was still in its primary school years, not nearly as trusted as today. Doctors also told Lynn that if she had the shunt, she wouldn't be a candidate later on for a transplant. It was one or the other. But now shunts were not an unsolvable surgical problem, and Klintmalm's plan was to take out the shunt as he did the transplant and to reconnect all the plumbing.

Money was another complication, as it is for most transplant patients. Sick for so long, Lynn had lost her group health insurance. She was too young for Medicare, too well-off for Medicaid, and caught in a generational trap on Social Security disability. Until her husband died, she could not qualify for disability benefits because she had never worked outside the home. It seemed ironic to her, amid a presidential campaign centered on "family values," that she found herself among a generation of fifty-something mothers and homemakers who did exactly what the "family values" crowd wanted them to do and then found themselves cut off from a Social Security program that paid disability benefits only to people who had worked for pay, outside the home. Another woman in her evaluation group still had a living husband, had never worked, and thus could not qualify for Social Security disability. Without that, she had no way to pay for a transplant at Baylor. She'd gone home to Oklahoma, perhaps to die.

The only insurance Lynn had been able to buy was a policy that paid no more than $50,000. Baylor requires patients to prove they have enough insurance or government assistance to cover the $150,000 minimum bill. If not, the patient has to put down cash in advance just to get on the waiting list. The files of patients who couldn't qualify financially and were sent home without hope would reach from floor to ceiling and beyond. Offering a transplant to all would bankrupt the program, hospital officials say.

"It's like asking Holiday Inn to house all the homeless," went the commonly quoted refrain.

For Lynn, whose husband, Bill, had been a fairly successful oil and watercolor artist, as well as a cartoonist for the *Saturday Evening Post*, that meant liquidating most of her retirement investments and writing a check to Baylor for $100,000.

"That was very frightening, to write a check for $100,000 to get a liver," she said.

It was a difficult choice, yet it seemed simple enough. There was no point in retirement money if you're dead. But it made the question all the more real: How much is the gamble at life worth? How much is it worth for two more years? Five more years? Ten more years?

It's the same question that the national debate on the high cost of health care boils down to. Officious terms float around the debate, but what the politicians, insurance companies, doctors, patients, employers, and everyone else are debating, is how much is a human life worth. What will society pay to keep someone alive or just to give a chance at staying alive? As the cost of transplanting escalates, and the cost of health care and health insurance becomes a bigger national issue, that question may someday have to be answered.

Now Lynn's mind was drifting to her surgical sister, her roulette partner, Mrs. Contreras. "This is so hard," she said.

Do you hope she dies? Do you hope you get the liver? Lynn began rooting for Yolanda Contreras as if the stranger were her own daughter.

The surgery began because Klintmalm couldn't say no to the family, couldn't find an iron-clad reason *not* to give it a try. Yolanda Contreras would get a chance. But her name was listed on the transplant board in Klintmalm's office with a question mark.

At 3:30 P.M., five hours after surgery began for Yolanda Contreras, Klintmalm called the nursing supervisor on the fourteenth floor from the operating room a dozen stories below to send the backup home. Klintmalm and Baylor's anesthesia chief, Mike Ramsay, who has pioneered some crucial advances in transplant surgery and has a huge national reputation himself, had "worked their magic."

"The case went along like any normal case," said Dr. Dale Distant, a surgeon from New York on a fellowship under Klintmalm.

13

"I'll be praying for the other woman," Lynn told Kathy O'Dea, who delivered the news. "I want to make sure I'm still on the list, that I haven't missed my chance, missed my turn."

"No, you're still on the list."

Weeks later, when a liver for Arden Lynn had not yet been found and Yolanda Contreras was still lying in a coma in the intensive care unit, neurologically worse than before the transplant and rejecting the transplanted liver on top of that, Goran Klintmalm was asked to second-guess himself.

"Maybe we should not have done her," he sighed. "There are no easy answers."

■

CHAPTER 2
THE DOCTORS

Not so many years ago, cardiologists were the pinnacle of the medical pyramid. Young kids in medical school who were the best of the best wanted to be the next Paul Dudley White. Cardiology progressed to cardiac surgery—cleaning out aortas, hooking up bypasses, even opening up the heart and making repairs. You were among the elite as a surgeon, but if you were a heart surgeon, you were something special, the cream of the crop, the top dog in the hospital cafeteria. It was the highest high-profile area of medicine, and the advances had been astounding: installing artificial valves, implanting pacemakers, replacing clogged arteries. Anybody could take out a gall bladder. Only the best could take apart a heart and put it back together. That got you on the cover of *Time* magazine.

Today, the "top gun" flyers of medicine are transplant surgeons, people who take bodies apart and remake them with somebody else's organs to save a life. It is the brave new world of health care, fraught with complications, ethical questions, incredible cost, and hope. Today, transplant surgeons are the pioneers of medicine, exploring and making up new rules as they go along. Now the most daring and gutsy cutters want to be transplant specialists—the next Barnard or DeBakey or Cooley or Shumway or Starzl. It is one of the youngest areas of medicine and one of the most rapidly advancing, venturing once again into the unknown world of transplanting animal organs into humans. It is the final frontier not yet conquered. Perhaps more than biotechnology and even genetic engineering, transplanting organs offers the most hope for yielding cures to previously fatal diseases. By definition, transplantation is a field that defies the laws of nature.

More than skill and brains perhaps, what it takes to be a good transplant surgeon is ego—enough of it to have the confidence to dismantle what nature conjured and try to do it better yourself. Imagine the gall of it all—tampering with creation, playing God. Transplant surgeons have brought a car mechanic's mentality to medicine: Need a new liver? We'll get you one. Would you like a new kidney while we're in there?

As astounding as its successes have been, transplantation still struggles for acceptance from society, for understanding, for support, both ethically and financially. It is governed by one simple, strange law: Life follows death. Someone must die so that someone may live. On top of the stress of dealing with someone's death comes the added burden of deciding which person among many will get the chance to live. It can all be a very heavy burden.

In the world of transplant surgeons, there are no office hours and few planned nights off. Their grueling world is governed by tragedies that befall others. A motorcycle accident may mean a heart is available. A stroke may yield a liver and two kidneys. Organs have to be harvested—that's the term— quickly. And tragedy seems to run in spurts, never conveniently spaced out or allocated or scheduled. Transplant teams can go days, even weeks, sitting around idle, then get caught up in a bang-bang-bang marathon of middle-of-the-night dashes to Lear jets and bumpy "red-balling" ambulance rides with a Coleman cooler holding a six-pack of organs.

"I've lived my life that way, feast or famine," said Goran Klintmalm.

For most of his life, there have been no easy answers for

■

16

Goran Bo Gustaf Klintmalm. Professionally, the tough decisions always fall to him, like the one about Yolanda Contreras,
and in transplanting, the tough decisions crop up with regular-
ity. These days, they have been coming more and more often.
And the choices are getting harder and harder. Charting the
right course has personally been a challenging and gripping
adventure for Goran, pronounced "Yor-ANN" but
Americanized by some simply to "Yorn."

"We are stepping into tragedy every time, every time,"
Klintmalm says. With transplants, "you become humble about
life. You see that life is very precious and very fragile and you
don't need to do much wrong to end up in a coffin. You always
respect death."

Klintmalm, a forty-three-year-old Swede known worldwide in transplantation circles for his surgical skill and scientific brilliance, came to Denver in 1979 to work as a fellow
under Tom Starzl, the man who performed the world's first
liver transplant and pioneered most of the field's advances.
Klintmalm had been the protégé at Stockholm's prestigious
Karolinska Institute of Swedish surgeon Carl Groth, himself a
transplant pioneer. After two and a half years with Starzl,
Klintmalm returned to Sweden and completed his Ph.D. Then
a couple of years later, in 1984, Starzl called to ask the younger
doctor to come back and run a satellite program of the suddenly overcrowded Pittsburgh center. It would be in Dallas, the first
transplant program in the Southwest.

Quickly, in less than five years, Klintmalm built one of
the world's leading transplant programs at Baylor with a combination of technical excellence, political astuteness, and extra-
ordinary efficiency. When a paper is published from Dallas,
said Dr. Rudolf Pichlmayr, the prominent head of Germany's
transplant program at Hannover, "We say, 'Oh, it's from
Klintmalm, so it's absolutely correct.'" But Baylor's success
hinges on more than just adventures in medical journals or
success with a scalpel. Klintmalm is part fund-raiser, part

bureaucrat, part wheeler-dealer, part politician, part decision maker. As good as he is in the operating room, he proves equally adroit in the boardrooms.

His program now brings in millions in revenue for the hospital, a sizable portion of the total business Baylor does each year. His team transplants about one hundred and fifty livers and sixty kidneys a year. To expand, Baylor is actively seeking patients from Mexico and beyond. And to further its research, Klintmalm and Baylor's fund-raisers have begun coddling contributors for endowed chairs for transplant physicians, money that helps relieve them of their regular pressures to see patients and generate income in exchange for time in the laboratory.

Klintmalm also has brought recognition internationally as well as locally. He has been featured prominently on television and in the local newspaper, such as a "High Profile" story in the *Dallas Morning News* usually reserved for socialites, sports heroes, and money moguls. His program also took on special prominence in the community when the daughter of the Dallas Cowboys' legendary coach, Tom Landry, was diagnosed with liver cancer. Pregnant, Lisa Landry Childress delivered her baby, then immediately was listed for a liver. In two weeks, Klintmalm and the top surgeon under him, Dr. Robert Goldstein, had come up with a new liver that saved her life and sparked Christmas-time headlines.

At forty-three, Klintmalm is almost an old man in transplanting, part of the pioneering second generation of liver swappers. (There are now three generations.) He prides himself on "pushing the envelope," being the first to try this or the first to do that, and his contributions and breakthroughs have been copied around the world—treatments for liver cancer, surgical procedures, drug therapies for transplant patients, and even a couple of patented medical instruments for transplant operations. His program has been so successful—a one-year survival rate of eighty-seven percent, compared with seventy-four percent nationally even though critical cases are sent his way from smaller hospitals—that insurance companies have contracted with him to send their customers to Baylor, which also offers a minimum price tag of $150,000, about half of the cost of a liver at Starzl's Pittsburgh center.

Blond, trim, and stylish, the urbane Goran Klintmalm barely shows the wrinkles of worry that have accumulated in just a few years. He sports designer glasses and a European wardrobe. He loves opera and books and is a testament to the American dream, having turned his talent into a millionaire's lifestyle: fancy BMW 850, showpiece house in Dallas's most exclusive neighborhood, polo with the tycoons of business on the weekend.

When a Dallas newspaper asked Klintmalm how his epitaph should read, he quoted Robert Louis Stevenson: "Life is not a matter of holding good cards, but of playing a poor hand well."

He grew up in a middle class suburb of Stockholm, the oldest of four children born to a mother who worked as an instructor of teachers for the deaf and a father who ran a cafe. As a boy, he was hooked on American television, westerns like *Bonanza*, and studied Native Americans. Adroit with his hands, with long, slender fingers, he built dioramas of cities.

He left Sweden with his wife, Tina, and three sons in part because the political and economic system was too restrictive, and risk takers were not rewarded, unlike in America.

"I was thirty-four years old and was given a chance to set up and run a program on my own and see if my wings were able to carry me," Klintmalm said. "That challenge was immense, to see if I was good enough to do this."

There were other issues as well. Klintmalm was displeased with a Swedish system that meant someone could "work hard and get less pay after tax than a janitor at night. The system did not encourage people to do their best and produce. It treated the dodos just like anyone else. I didn't see any future there, and I wanted to be able to get my chance to try out."

Still, it was a tough call, taking his children from their heritage. Goran and Tina didn't want them to lose their Swedish culture and "get into the hamburger culture." Although the parents speak Swedish at home, the boys speak English among themselves. "We try to make it both European as well as American," he said.

Klintmalm can't imagine going back now. He would like to become an American citizen, but as a Swedish citizen, he would first have to renounce his citizenship there. "I think one day I will get to that point," he said, but not yet.

Like many of the early pioneers, Klintmalm became enamored with liver transplanting simply because it was so difficult, because many said it *couldn't* be done.

The liver is an unromantic organ, vital and yet obscure to most. Lovers don't carve their initials on trees inside the outline of a liver. Nobody attaches much soulful or spiritual relevance to the liver. Yet unlike the heart or the kidneys, there is still no way to compensate for lack of a liver. And surgically, transplanting a liver is far more difficult than doing a heart, even though hearts grab all the headlines. In the early days, even before Klintmalm arrived in Denver, liver transplanting was a marathon ordeal taking fifteen to twenty-five hours, with poor prospects for success and good potential for scorn. Most patients died, and no one died easily. They either bled to death all over the operating room table, or suffered slow, tortuous, painful demises from liver failure.

"Just because it was difficult. I wanted to see if I could do it," Klintmalm said.

He takes the same approach to running the Baylor program now. "The thing that distinguishes Klintmalm and this program is his unending desire to move ahead, his not being satisfied with state of the art, but taking it a step ahead. We're trying to push the art to its limit," said Goldstein, Klintmalm's assistant director, partner and, sometimes, alter ego.

If Hollywood called for another gorgeous-sidekick TV

doctor, a Robert Kiley to Marcus Welby, a Gonzo Gates to Trapper John, Bob Goldstein would be perfect for the role. With shoulder-length curly brown hair, now graying on the ends, boyish good looks and a black Lexus with pink fuzzy dice hanging from the rearview mirror, Goldstein was the doctor the nurses at Baylor Medical Center gossiped about for years until his recent marriage. He is, after all, at the top of the medical heap, able to charm with his skill and savvy, or just soften them with his eyes.

Bob Goldstein stories are legendary around Baylor. He came as a fellow—a doctor who has completed his internship and residency but undertakes a fellowship in a specialty before venturing out on his own in that area. Goldstein was one of Klintmalm's first fellows, and he stood out immediately: a long-haired, sandal-wearing Jew who threw the Baptist hospital administration into a tizzy.

"Dr. Goldstein, what about the dress code?"

"What dress code?"

"Dr. Goldstein, what about shoes?"

"What shoes?"

Goldstein's free-form casualness even carries over to his dining room, which might be considered, well, a work in progress. Unhappy with the walls, Goldstein one night bought some colorful tempera paints at a crafts store and offered his dinner guests the chance to paint. Since then, friends have been constantly painting and repainting, scribbling messages, sayings, and thoughts on the walls, now ablaze with frivolity.

"I told the wife when we got married, 'There are a lot of things you can change, but the dining room stays,'" laughs Goldstein, now forty.

For vacation, Bob Goldstein and his bride joined an expedition to climb Mount Everest and made it to 18,000 feet. Life just can't have enough thrills or challenges.

At Christmas, Klintmalm hosts a stylish, fancy Swedish glögg party for all the bigwigs at Baylor, including his

■

staff, fellow physicians, contributors, and friends. It is a warm, formal affair, famous for the strength of the glögg as well as the power people it attracts. And it is as socially correct as Goldstein's annual tree-decorating party, the "bush party," is socially incorrect. At the exceedingly casual Goldstein bash, friends bring an ornament for the Hanukkah bush, usually but not necessarily X-rated, and then a gift for a blind gift exchange. If nothing else, the two parties highlight the difference between the two men.

What saved Goldstein in strict, uptight Dallas was his surgical prowess. When working on a patient he dives in, almost climbing into the belly, a whiz of tying and cutting, almost as fast as Klintmalm himself. Goldstein appears to violate the patient's space in an almost intimate way, invading the body and blurring the line between the two people. He has little tolerance for mistakes by staff in the operating room. Like Klintmalm, he has crossed the four-hour barrier for completing a liver transplant. Then, to unwind, he often takes off on his bike for an eleven-mile ride around Dallas's White Rock Lake.

Unlike Klintmalm, Goldstein didn't set out to be a surgeon, didn't race after transplanting because it was the biggest challenge. He grew up in the eastern mountains of Tennessee, a child of the '60s and the son of a textile executive. He dropped out of the University of Tennessee after too many student demonstrations and too many bad grades and too much interest in women and fun. He would have flunked out after his first year if not for credits in photography and badminton. He came home to Elizabethton, Tennessee, and thought he might work in the plant his father ran. His mother was the personnel director.

"They said they would not give me a job unless I cut my hair, so I said, 'OK, I'm going back to Knoxville,'" Goldstein said. "Then Buford, my dad, decided it was best to keep me home. So he gave me a job dyeing carpet yarn, the worst job in the plant."

After working a three-to-eleven shift all summer walking huge racks of carpet yarn into and out of an oven and after befriending and listening to the old-time plant employees wise beyond their careers, Goldstein decided college wasn't so bad after all.

Buford, not convinced his young radical was serious, gave him one quarter to prove himself. He had been kicked out of the dorm for "total disregard for the rules," so he had to find his own apartment. Despite another run-in with the administration after he showed up wearing blue jeans, a T-shirt, and a ponytail for a prestigious reception at the president's house for the children of university contributors, Goldstein managed to stay on the honor roll every quarter.

But his was not the classic story of the driven student intent on medical school. Botany was Bob's passion, and he set off for a Ph.D. at Wisconsin, ready to become the world's expert on the origins of corn. When he got there, he didn't like the head of the program, so he turned around and went home to Tennessee.

On the spur of the moment, facing his parents who, at the least, had not expected to see him back on the doorstep so soon, Bob suddenly said he had decided to go into medicine. Actually, it was about all he could think of that might get them off his back. He got a job as an orderly at a Knoxville hospital, took classes in the afternoon, and landed at Tennessee's medical school in Memphis.

Pediatrics was his chosen career, but his residency in Ohio proved too boring, so pediatric surgery seemed like the thing to do. He spent two years as a general surgical resident in Morgantown, West Virginia, and then another year as a researcher in pediatric surgery at Johns Hopkins. He thought he had landed a pediatric surgical fellowship in Pittsburgh.

■

"The guy in Pittsburgh said there had been a mixup, and there wasn't a spot for me that year, but Tom Starzl owed him some favors, and why don't I do transplants for a year then come back to pediatrics," he said.

"I went there to see what it was like, and I sat in the office in a chair forever. No one talked to me. It was a mess, typical Pittsburgh."

Soon he received a call from Starzl's office to report to Dallas for three months beginning July 1, 1985. The new program there needed help.

"They said get hold of this guy 'Klintmalm.' Clint-what? I'd never heard of him. Nobody had ever heard of him. Nobody knew what Baylor was. They'd heard of UCLA, Nebraska and Pittsburgh—that's it.

"Klintmalm said, 'We'd be glad to have you come down for six months. . . .'

"Six months! Here it goes again, the jack-around."

When he arrived, never having done or seen a transplant, Bob Goldstein was the only fellow at the time. Soon he was asked to stay a full year, but before that time was up, Klintmalm wanted to make him a partner.

"Starzl got miffed, I heard. He said, 'I recruited that boy myself.' Hah! He never saw me.

"I really got into it, I think, because it is the only frontier in medicine left.

"I get off on seeing somebody who ought to be belly up walk out of here and come back a year later. Most of them come back and they're excited about life, excited to have a second chance."

CHAPTER 3
THE SWITCH

To say it had been a hard week around the transplant unit would be like saying the "reelection thing" didn't go well for George Bush. Actually, it had been hell. A woman recently transplanted had "crashed and burned" inexplicably, first having seizures, then looking as if she had an infection, except that nothing grew in cultures or tests. She "circled the drain" for a few days in the intensive care unit, then died. An autopsy found nothing wrong, except that she was dead. "It's still a mystery, a big mystery," Klintmalm said.

Even harder to swallow, though, was the death of Bobby Murray, a well-liked, outgoing African-American police officer from Washington, D.C., who had been retransplanted at Baylor. His wife and three-year-old daughter, who came to know many of the doctors by first name, had become favorites with the transplant team and with the other patients. In better days, Murray had visited patients to offer encouragement and humor. His wife had been a pillar of strength through a long ordeal. His daughter teased the four surgical fellows on the transplant team, especially Dr. Lars Backman from Sweden, who had a daughter the same age.

But in the last week, Bobby Murray's heart had just about given out, his lungs were barely functioning, his immune system was attacking his liver—a process called rejection—sending out killer cells to destroy the foreign tissue. On top of that, his bile duct was leaking, and his belly was full of infection. "Why do I have such a burden?" Murray's wife wondered aloud one day.

There is no answer. If you ask a theologian, "Why?," the best answer may be simply, "Because."

"It pains me every time I see his family," Klintmalm said that week during rounds. "It's like his primary coverage is with Murphy's Law."

Bending at the waist over Murray's bed, Goran Klintmalm, world-class surgeon, healer and pioneer, buried his head in his hands one day in a moment of silence.

"He has a lung problem, a heart problem, a kidney problem, a liver problem, a sepsis problem, a wound problem, and he may have a neurological problem. Virtually every system has a problem."

Then he stood up, threw his hands in the air, as if looking for guidance from gods of higher authority, and wondered out loud, oblivious to the team standing behind him:

"What can we do? What can we do?"

The next day, Klintmalm sat down with Murray's wife to discuss invoking his living will and pulling the plug, while coordinators babysat the three-year-old. The life support disconnected, a heart monitor was turned on in the central nurses' station of the intensive care unit. On rounds, most of the team kept staring at its erratic waves, waiting for the moment. By the time the team reached the fourteenth floor, a phone call came to the nurses' station for Klintmalm. He turned to Thomas Gonwa, the widely respected kidney expert at Baylor. "Tom, can you start rounds? Bobby Murray just expired," he announced to the team, thirty minutes after the plug was pulled.

To save their sanity, most members of the team made a point of not getting close to the patients, because they never know which ones will live and which ones will die. Yet as hardened to life-and-death dramas as they had become, as thick-

■

skinned and protective of their own sanity as they had grown, as sure of the outcome as they had been for more than a week now, Bobby Murray's death was a deep blow. "It seems like the nice people never get a break," nurse Janel McDonald sighed. "I know that's not rational, but it always seems true."

On Wednesday, the day after Bill Clinton ousted George Bush from the presidency, Swedish citizen Goran Klintmalm decided his staff needed some levity, some fun, a laugh to ease the pain and tension of the grim, emotionally draining week. GK walked into the office that morning with a "gimme" cap on, pants pulled up almost to his armpits, and a pocket protector in his shirt over his breast. "Howdy, all. I'm from Ark-Can-Sarwwwww," he squealed in a nerdy, piggish voice. "I'm from Ark-Can-Sarwwwwwwwwwwwwwwwwwwww."

It was just what the doctor ordered. "Did you hear what GK did this morning?" the chatter went. "Can you believe what GK did this morning? He's from Ark-Can-Sarw!" they laughed.

Humor for Klintmalm is important, both for the staff and the patients. "If I'm laughing, things can't be all that grim," he says. One time he turned to a high-strung patient, who was in the middle of a long, hard battle with rejection. At the moment, the patient was freaking out over the news that one drug was not working and another would have to be tried. Klintmalm stared him right in the eye with a severity only a doctor delivering terrible news could muster. "Jack," Klintmalm stated in his compassionate, yet oh-so-serious tone, "don't ever play poker with your own money."

One day after the "Ar-Can-Sawr" joke, Goran Klintmalm found himself up most of the night, again. He and one of his surgical fellows, Dr. Caren Eisenstein, had arrived at Dallas Love Field at 1:30 A.M. for a short flight to Tyler, Texas, only seventy miles or so to the east. They waited for the Southwest Organ Bank to line everything up, then took off in a large, wide Westwind private jet, a "flying bathtub," Eisenstein dubbed it, in unseasonable cold weather. It was 3:30 A.M. by the time they reached Memorial Hospital in Tyler, and then they waited and waited and waited because they couldn't find anyone to help, even anyone to direct them to the proper locker room to change into scrubs.

The family of the fifty-eight-year-old stroke victim had specified that no harvesting surgery could last past 7 A.M. so the body could be prepared for a quick burial. As a result, the organ bank had opted only to place the liver, making Klintmalm's work faster and easier. Or so he thought. The man turned out to have abnormal anatomy—a hepatic artery in a place where it shouldn't be. If a mistake is made in the retrieval of the organ, it can be lost. But Klintmalm became suspicious early when he could feel a pulse—though brain dead, the man's heart still beat while on life support equipment—back behind the liver where one shouldn't be. His detective work saved the liver.

It was 7 A.M. when Klintmalm and Eisenstein landed at Love Field, greeted by the first frost of the year. Eisenstein scraped her windshield with a cassette tape; Klintmalm with a credit card. Eisenstein asked him if the cold reminded him of Sweden, if he still liked the cold. No, too much Texan in him now. He didn't like the cold at all.

Back at Baylor, Klintmalm found himself again holding the reins of grief. The liver from Tyler was first to be for a sixty-seven-year-old Swiss scientist, Eugene Konecci, who had worked with Wernher von Braun in the early days of the American rocketry program and had been an early pioneer in the National Aeronautics and Space Administration. Konecci, a medical doctor with a Ph.D., reminded the Swedish M.D.s and Ph.D.s of themselves, and everyone who met him agreed he was one of the nicest, brightest people who had every come through evaluation at Baylor. He had contracted hepatitis years before, probably drawing blood samples from astronauts during the experimental "Right Stuff" days of the space race. The hepatitis C had slowly destroyed his liver, and now cancer had invaded.

■

The selection committee, which meets every Wednesday at Baylor, is made up of internal medicine physicians, the transplant surgeons, cardiologists, cancer specialists, social workers, and even the chaplain (as a nonvoting member). The group instantly fell in love with Gene Konecci—a contemporary, one of their own. He had two strikes against him, however. For twenty-five years the hepatitis C had been working away on his liver, and it was now shot. More threatening was the cancer. Liver cancer is one of the most deadly strains of this killer, generally considered incurable. It kills quickly in most cases, either rapidly spreading to other organs from the liver, or exponentially growing inside the liver, then rupturing it, killing the patient almost instantly from blood loss. In the early days of liver transplantation, there was great hope that by removing the liver with the tumor, a patient could be "cured" of liver cancer. Then, doctors discovered that the tumors recur either because microscopic cancerous cells were left behind, or because the cancer is triggered by something else—a virus perhaps or a cancer strain hidden somewhere else in the body. This finding actually opens new doors to the understanding of cancer, but it also prompted some transplant centers to restrict offering new livers to cancer patients.

Klintmalm and a transplant surgeon in Paris, France, are the two notable exceptions who had not given up on treating liver cancer through transplants. At Baylor, Klintmalm has developed a chemotherapy and transplant plan—a "protocol"—that includes doses of chemotherapy in the operating room. It has generated a five-year survival rate of fifty percent, magnitudes better than any other transplant center in the world, and better than any other chemotherapy or liver cancer treatment so far. It has become one of his pet obsessions, and Klintmalm has also begun building an international computer registry for liver transplants for cancer. His protocol has recently begun to be adopted by other centers as well.

To be accepted into Klintmalm's cancer experiment,

one has to arrive at Baylor before the tumor spreads beyond the liver. Any cancer elsewhere in the body will take off and grow like mesquite bushes once the patient's immune system is suppressed to prevent rejection of the new organ. So a transplant for somebody with cancer somewhere else in the body only speeds death. Once accepted into the program, cancer patients receive priority on the waiting list.

In Gene Konecci's case, a magnetic resonance imaging test revealed suspicious signs that the cancer had spread. The committee agonized over the finding, finally concluding that he was such a "nice guy" that he deserved the benefit of the doubt. Konecci, a consultant and professor at the University of Texas at Austin, would be put on the list if his insurance company would agree to pay for the transplant and chemotherapy. As with all cancer patients, his surgery would have to be done with a backup ready. There is no way to be sure whether the cancer has spread until the surgeons open the abdomen, take tissue samples to the lab, feel around with their own fingers, and look with their own eyes.

It took the University of Texas health system four weeks to make up its mind, finally agreeing to pay for the transplant. Now, at last, Konecci was approved and a liver was available. While GK had been in Tyler, Konecci and his wife drove to Dallas from Austin and he was prepped for surgery in room 35.

Melvin Berg was the quintessential Florida entrepreneur until he became too sick to work. After raising a family of five in Chicago as a plumber, a barkeep, and an automobile salesman/dealer, Berg "retired" early to Miami, in 1971, where he soon found himself tinkering with golf clubs. He had always been handy, a restless repairman of Scandinavian descent who wanted to fix, or improve, just about everything he saw. Golf clubs—he could make them better. Put on a new shaft, a better grip, adjust the driver this way or that way. Soon he was repairing clubs for pro shops at southern Florida's plethora of country clubs. Next he was building entire sets of clubs for friends, and *their* friends, and *their* friends. Want a set of Pings, copies of Pings, for one-third the cost? Call my friend Mel. Berg's following spread so far that he built special clubs for Miami Dolphin's quarterbacks Dan Marino and Don Strock. "I had a pretty good business going until I got sick," he said.

Berg was sixty-seven years old, although he looked ten, maybe twenty, years younger. Lanky and trim, he dashed around with a mop of white hair, walking every day to stay fit. He knew he was old but didn't feel it until fatigue and nausea suddenly set in, and fluid began accumulating in his belly. He ended up with an esteemed gastroenterologist in Miami who diagnosed him with cholangitis in his liver—the bile ducts were scarred and diseased, thus bile was clogging his liver, rendering it increasingly unable to power the rest of the body. A couple of experimental drug treatments were tried—with no success. Finally, Berg was told his only hope was a liver transplant. Miami had a liver transplant program, but Berg wasn't thrilled with the one-year survival rate of sixty-eight percent. Besides, Medicare had not yet agreed to pay for patients in Miami. The government agency will pay for transplants only at approved "Centers of Excellence." Berg learned that Baylor in Dallas was approved for Medicare and had a one-year survival rate of eighty-seven percent. Besides, he had a daughter who lived in a Dallas suburb.

At sixty-seven, some might not want to endure an ordeal like a liver transplant, eight hours or so of grueling surgery, three months of difficult recovery, emotional and physical ups and downs, and a lifetime of drugs that bring with them a host of side effects. In essence, one disease is traded for another, and statistically, the elderly do not tolerate it all nearly as well as younger patients. Berg didn't know it, but Baylor's one-year survival rate for people over sixty-five was closer to fifty percent.

■

"I'll be dead in a year without this transplant. And maybe it will prolong my life three years, five years or so. So I'll pick up an extra two or three years," he said with classic Midwestern matter-of-factness. "But my quality of life is zero now. I can't live the way I want to live. I don't have the energy to live. I look at this as just something that has to be done."

What's more, in the climate of health-care reform and skyrocketing costs and insurance premiums, a tough public-policy question was hanging over the heads of people like Berg. Is society able to pay for transplants for those over sixty-five, especially in an environment of organ shortages? So far, Americans have been willing. Other countries have not, imposing age cutoffs for expensive, daring medical treatments. Berg's transplant would cost the taxpayers a minimum of $150,000. Will the day come when the United States decides that the benefit is not worth the cost, that the money—and the donated liver—should go to someone younger? Luckily for Mel Berg, there is no age cutoff for transplants—for now. The fallout from health-care reform will eventually be rationing of expensive treatments, and age is one simple way to ration.

By the time Berg arrived at Baylor in June, his size nine feet had swelled to size thirteen, and his weight had shot up from 180 to 204. He couldn't walk one block, and he could barely breathe on his own, so much fluid had pooled inside his body. Harry Sarles, one of Baylor's gastroenterologists (internal medicine physicians who specialize in digestive diseases, including liver ailments) checked Berg into the hospital immediately. Sarles improved his nutrition, drained four liters of liquid from his lungs, and tapped his belly to relieve it of the ascites.

"Sarles really fixed me up good," Berg said. "Then I got real skinny."

Berg's weight dropped to 155, and he was evaluated for a transplant. Although there was increasing concern at Baylor about the potential for older patients and apprehension about a

■

possible ballooning of Berg's portal vein that could cause a complication in surgery, he was accepted in July and told the wait had grown from a couple of weeks to a month or two.

"We thought we'd be here eight weeks," Berg said in November, after buying winter clothes for the first time in two decades. "I've got to get on with my life if there is going to be one."

The wait was wearing on him. Nervous about being forgotten, or becoming too sick for the transplant before the call came, Berg called Baylor weekly to check on his status, clung tightly to his beeper, and pushed himself to walk at least a mile daily to stay in the best physical shape possible. "The last couple of weeks have really gotten to be a drag now. You come to a point where you want to say, 'The hell with it. Forget it.' You know? First they said eight weeks, then twelve weeks, and twelve weeks came and went. Now I'm here seventeen weeks. Sarles's nurse said seventeen weeks is the record, nobody goes over that, so I'll be in soon. I hope she's right."

Three days later, November 5, Mel Berg got the call. Actually, his daughter got the call. He had been lying in bed, awakened by the rustlings of two grandchildren getting ready for school. His daughter, Cathy, came into the room at 7 A.M.

"It looks like today may be the day. They want you down there as a backup," Cathy said.

"If it is, OK, so be it," Berg told Cathy. "But I hope the other guy makes it. It's bad enough one person has to die to get a liver. Now two have to go for me to get it."

The fourteenth floor was completely full by the time Mel Berg arrived at Baylor. The suite normally used for prepping patients was occupied by the family of another transplant to be performed that day, this one with a liver of rare AB blood type flown in from Atlanta. That operation had been hurried to start at 5 A.M. to free the operating room for the second transplant—

■

Konecci's—which would follow. Overnight, Gene Konecci had checked into the last empty room on the fourteenth floor. So Berg was asked to wait in the easy chairs by the elevators until Klintmalm decided whether the cancer patient would get the liver, or not.

By now sixty-eight years old, Berg was nonchalant. His wife, Connie, and daughter came down to Baylor with him, but he was convinced this was only a dry run. He didn't want to call his other four children and excite them—no need for them to start scrambling for plane reservations into Dallas or anything.

Like Arden Lynn, Berg began cheering for the "other guy"—the cancer patient whose name he did not know. Statistically, he had been told, most backups do not get the liver, but they appreciated his coming down because they just have to make sure that a liver never goes to waste. In the past eight years of the Baylor program, "I can think of only a handful of times when the surgery didn't go through," chaplain Grady Hinton told Berg.

"Mr. Berg. Can you come talk to Sharon Carlen on the phone?" A nurse summoned Berg to the front desk on the floor, to talk with one of the transplant team coordinators.

"They are going to abort the transplant, and you'll get the liver," Carlen told Berg.

"What do I do?"

"Stay there. We have to get you ready FAST. Is your family there?"

"Yes."

At the same time, Klintmalm's distinctive and resonant European voice popped up at the nurses' station. Nurses began yelling. Activity went instantly into overdrive. Kathy O'Dea soon was barking orders.

Klintmalm saw Berg, stopped him, said something briefly, and then continued on. Berg walked slowly back towards his wife, his skin, usually jaundiced from his liver dis-

■

ease, now as pale as his white hair. He forced a weak "thumbs up" sign.

"I'm going. They want me now," he said, as Connie Berg instantly, silently, broke into tears.

Berg had to be prepped as soon as possible. The liver had been without blood for about twelve hours now, and even though preservation fluid keeps it viable for eighteen hours, Berg faced more than an hour for the emergency surgical prep, followed by several hours to remove his liver and prepare the donor liver for transplant. Time was growing short, and the operating room staff, tired from the morning transplant and depressed at having aborted Gene Konecci's surgery, was ready to end the day's work.

But first there was a problem on the fourteenth floor—there was no room available for Berg. Kathy O'Dea moved Mrs. Konecci out of her husband's room, number 35, ordering it cleaned and readied for the new patient.

Klintmalm headed straight for Mrs. Konecci, first taking her to O'Dea's office to deliver the bad news. The cancer had spread to the stomach, piercing the gastrohepatic tissue, the plane that separates the stomach and the liver. There was nothing that could be done. He was very sorry. But they tried, and that's all that could be done. The grieving widow-to-be then was shepherded into a "family room," a tiny, windowless, dark closet outfitted with Bibles and Kleenex boxes where relatives are taken to cry over bad news out of sight of the other patients and families.

Dr. Tom Renard, another of Klintmalm's four fellows, was in charge of prepping Berg. "What's the patient's name?" he hurriedly yelled to the nurses' station.

"B-i-r-g? B-u-r-g? B-e-r-g? What's the first name?"

"Dr. Renard, what's the skin time on Mr. Berg?" a nurse yelled, referring to the time scheduled for the operation to begin—the opening of the skin.

■

"ASAP."

It was a scene of chaos, organized chaos if there can be such a thing. Klintmalm told Renard he wanted to start on Berg right away. "I want to get this done soon," he said glumly, obviously upset about Konecci. The operating room had fallen silent when the declaration was made, pierced with soft cries of "Oh, shit" from those assisting Klintmalm. "It was pretty grim in there," said Dr. Dale Distant, another of the four fellows. "What can you do?" There are few bigger disappointments in transplanting than to abort, sew someone back up and send the patient home to die.

At the same time, Klintmalm had another patient to deal with, a long-time patient who had been told that day that her third liver was failing and she would need a fourth liver— her third transplant. She cornered Klintmalm in the hallway, put her head on his shoulder and cried. Mrs. Konecci walked by, crying, leaving the claustrophobic family room for a "day treatment" room—little more than an examination table—that had more light in it.

Klintmalm wanted some six hours of preparations on Berg to be done in forty-five minutes or so. A portable X-ray machine whizzed down the hall to room 35, an anesthesiologist hurried in to take a complete history, a "vampire"—a technician who draws blood—came in to fill twenty-five tubes with Berg's blood.

"My blood pressure's way up," Berg said. "I'm nervous." He was shaking. He had no idea he was lying in the same bed in which Gene Konecci had been prepped a few hours before.

At 4:15 P.M., Gene Konecci's name was still on the white board in Klintmalm's office where transplants are posted. And an orderly showed up to take Berg down to the second-floor operating room on a gurney.

"I love you," he said to his daughter and wife.

"You can go down with him," another patient told Mrs. Berg. She ran after the stretcher.

■

Berg, at the elevators, spotted Grady Hinton, the chaplain, and stopped him, asking for a prayer.

Hinton, who was on his way to console the woman told she'll need a third transplant, was spinning in the vortex of confusion and grief as well. The elevator behind him, held open by the orderly, began a steady alarm: "Bong. Bong. Bong." Hinton quickly oriented himself to Berg and grabbed his hand.

"We pray for this life-giving transplant, Father," the elevator punctuating the invocation with its incessant "Bong." "We pray for family, for the doctors and nurses and technicians . . ." Bong. Bong. Bong.

After Berg was wheeled down to O.R. 4, his daughter wandered out to the waiting area by the elevators where the family had spent most of the day. Mrs. Konecci, too, was sitting there, waiting for her husband to come up from the recovery room. Neither knew who the other was. Neither spoke.

"I couldn't really talk to either, and I needed to talk to both," Hinton said. "It was strange to have them bumping into each other. To not get the transplant is the toughest thing in some ways. You're all prepared for a miracle, expecting a miracle, and it doesn't happen and you're left with no hope suddenly. It's the biggest swing of emotion we see."

Later, Berg's daughter Cathy, back in room 35 visiting with Hinton, told her mother she was going back to the elevators to sit.

"I said, 'I don't know any other way to tell you this except very honestly. That's the wife of the other patient sitting by the elevator. I think it's best if you not go out there,'" Hinton said.

"She thanked me and said she understood. It's very unfortunate we didn't have a room for the wife. I think maybe we need to put these people on separate floors. I was very afraid they'd strike up a conversation."

Grady Hinton went home that night and slumped on the couch silently. "What's wrong with you?" his wife asked.

■

"That was one of the hardest days I've had in years. It was as chaotic as I've ever seen," he said. "I'm very concerned about how we do these things. There were some very awkward, uncomfortable situations."

Twelve floors below, Mel Berg was laid out on the altar that is the operating room table, his arms extended to each side and strapped down as if on the cross. Cellophane bags were placed over his arms—like children's water wings—and warm air was pumped in to help maintain his body temperature in the sometimes chilly room. Needles were inserted into his veins, and anesthetic drugs were quickly pumped in, knocking him out in seconds. His chest was shaved with a Bic disposable razor, then washed with disinfectant and swabbed with dark orange germ-killer. Over all that, Berg was draped in aqua-blue paper of the consistency of cloth. At vital junctions, blue towels were stapled to his skin, as if the patient had become a piece of plywood. Electrodes stuck to his chest to monitor his heart. Needles attached to tubes and bags of fluid ran into his neck and his arm and to a machine called "Cell Saver," which collects blood from the "suckers" surgeons use to drain bloody areas, then purifies it, stokes it with some helpful nutrients and returns it to the patient's body, reducing the need for transfusions. Everything was covered, except for a bread-box-sized square of flesh illuminated under a foursome of fierce bright lights. It was as if the humanity of the patient was completely covered, perhaps for the sanity of the physicians as well as the sterility of the procedure, and what was before the surgeons on the table was a machine to be fixed. It's very easy to forget that there is a father and husband under all the covering.

"Chris, can we start?" Dale Distant asked anesthesiology fellow Chris Hellman.

"Yes, please."

Tonight, Distant would be the lead surgeon, assisted by

■

Klintmalm and by a general surgeon who scrubbed in to be "second assistant" on the transplant. There are always three surgeons—the attending, who is always Klintmalm or one of his trio of staff transplant surgeons, plus a transplant fellow and a "support surgeon" called in from a list of Baylor doctors who like to assist on transplants.

For Distant, this was the third liver for which he had been the lead surgeon "skin to skin"—opening to closing. A New York native, father of three, including twin three-year-olds, and husband of a Veterans Administration hospital nurse, the thirty-two-year-old tall, balding African-American surgeon had already done a fellowship in kidney transplants and now had come to spend a year with Klintmalm. He was near the top of the medical pinnacle and was rapidly excelling—even though he was making only $30,000 a year. Distant surprised even Klintmalm on some days with insightful and wise diagnoses and suggestions. Surgically, his hands were very skilled. Personally, the patients took an immediate liking to his straightforward answers, calm manner, and friendly demeanor.

Now he moved a scalpel down Mel Berg's stomach and then reached for the "Bovie."

The Bovie is to the surgeon what the bow is to the violinist. It looks like an old-style electric toothbrush, a piece of plastic with an on-off switch a thumb's length from the end and a pointed tip. When the switch is pushed, electric current twitches through the tip of the Bovie, cutting by burning and cauterizing at the same time. Better than a scalpel because it stops bleeding as it cuts, the Bovie is the knife of choice for surgeons now. When the tip collects blackened goo, it is simply scraped across a Brillo-like pad.

The Bovie's only byproduct is smell, a putrid odor of burned flesh, blackened blood, and incinerated wet tissue that temporarily turns the operating room into a place of sickening stench that must be something like a cremation furnace. The smell lasts briefly—air-circulation fans clean it out quickly. But to visitors, the most unsettling part of observing surgery is not the sight but the smell.

Distant cut straight down Berg's chest then went off at forty-five degree angles toward each side, making an incision shaped like an upside down Y or a Mercedes Benz emblem. The technique, in fact, is called a Mercedes incision, and it leaves liver transplant patients with a car logo permanently scarred on their bellies. When the incision was complete, Distant pulled each side of the chest wall up and out, peeling back the slabs to expose Berg's belly.

The inside of the human abdomen looks like a perfectly packed suitcase—each organ, each piece of tissue, filling its specified spot with no wasted space and yet no wrinkles from overpacking. In this case, the suitcase was about to be unpacked and then repacked with someone else's pants. At first glance, the placement of the insides can look chaotic and random, but on more careful observation, order emerges from the jumble. Squiggles and blocks, rounds and squares, balance each other and form an artistic beauty—Matisse cutouts balanced and juxtaposed to form a masterpiece of radiance. Forms appear carefully crafted for a specific purpose, colors are balanced and pleasing to the eye. There could be no finer example of nature's aesthetic wonder.

Berg, GK noted to Distant, has a mitral valve prolapse in his heart—where the valve has fallen down on the job—which necessitated special attention. And he has a possible portal vein thrombosis—an enlargement of the vein that carries blood away from the liver. Because of a weak spot in the vein wall, it puffs up much like a balloon when air is first blown in. If there is a thrombosis, Distant will have to work out some special routing of Berg's new portal vein. "We may have to go past the pancreas," Klintmalm said, "to find a place for the anastomosis"—the spot where the donor end is tied to the recipient end of a vessel.

The mood was somber as the third patient of the day

■

was opened in O.R. 4. "It's the nice guys who never get a break," the support surgeon, Dr. Miller Bell, suggested, referring to Gene Konecci. "You can have a drug-using, HIV-positive hemophiliac burglar get hit by a truck and not a scratch. But nice guys don't stand a chance."

Klintmalm tried to brighten spirits as he cupped a lapful of intestines with his hands so that Distant could cut with the Bovie inside. He began kidding with nurses, razzing them about the location of instruments, and joking with the anesthesia team.

As Distant probed, burned, and tied off Berg's insides, Klintmalm taught, showing a technique here, a pointer there. "You have to be cautious here," he suggested. "That's right. That's right."

Berg's liver looked shrunken, all pimply, and stiff as a pencil eraser. White, fat-like knobs clustered on the outside of the liver, a result of the cholangitis inside. Distant found the hepatic artery, which did have a thrombosis, and then moved down toward the portal vein, which Klintmalm found and pointed out to him. The dissection—trimming the liver out of its longtime home, like carving a pumpkin and then taking the lid off—is a hunt, finding the right vessels through touch, sight, experience, and a bit of guesswork.

"This guy really is in good shape for his age. That should make it easier," Klintmalm suggested.

Suddenly blood spurted up from Berg, spraying the surgeons with fine droplets. A hole was punctured in the vena cava when the adrenal vein was tied off.

Klintmalm leaned in, trying to plug the hole with his fingers. Blood was pouring out of Berg now, the suckers trying to keep up as bright red fluid was carried off to the Cell Saver.

Distant quickly stitched in under Klintmalm's finger and up the other side of the tiny hole. Quickly, he had it closed.

"A little hole in the vena cava has been plugged. That's all," Klintmalm declared loudly in a singsong voice.

■

"Well, I'll just give him a little more fluid," Chris Hellman offered casually.

"It wasn't fluid he was losing," Klintmalm deadpanned. "It was blood."

If anything, the episode showed how far the art of liver transplantation has come. A patient undergoing a liver transplant, perhaps the most difficult and involved of all major surgeries, can bleed uncontrollably, requiring hundreds of units of blood to be rapidly infused if there is to be any hope of survival. Patients in liver failure usually lack the normal blood clotting mechanisms the liver provides, so it's very hard to stop the bleeding. In the early days of transplanting, when the procedures were not as refined and took much longer and the equipment and techniques were not as advanced, cities feared that a transplant could drain the entire blood bank in one night.

"When the program was going to get started here, nobody on the anesthetic side wanted anything to do with it," said Mike Ramsay, the Baylor chief of anesthesiology who is now considered one of the best in the world at transplant anesthesia. "They had heard about the long, all-night procedures with Starzl, and the bad outcomes. They could be a horrendous, time-consuming bloodbath."

When the Cell Saver device came on the market, Ramsay says, Pittsburgh published a paper questioning its use in transplants because they had had terrible results with it. Ramsay, on the other hand, made the device work by developing a way to insert blood-clotting factors as the Cell Saver washed blood. His technique has now been adopted by other transplant programs—one of many innovations out of Baylor. Another is a Stat-Lab located around the corner from O.R. 4 which can give the anesthesiologist laboratory readings on the patient's blood in as little as sixty seconds, giving the operating room an almost instant assessment of the patient's condition. "We can go much closer to the edge because we know we can get lab values back within a minute," Ramsay says.

■

As Berg's surgery progressed, and thoughts wandered to what a wild day it had been, the chatter over his belly turned to more important topics, like the musical selections in O.R. 4. The radio was turned to one of those "Lite Rock" stations with sappy love songs, the kind that almost always seem to include the line, *"I couldn't help myself. . . ."* Tired and a bit bored, the scrub nurse declared the music terrible and asked for something more appropriate. "What do you want, rap?" GK asked.

"No," the African-American nurse said. "Something nice and jazzy."

Klintmalm chose for a compact disc, "Moondance," which set the anesthesiologist dancing.

"We have a Van Morrison fan here," Klintmalm said. "I just bought his latest."

Depending on his mood, Klintmalm chooses anything from classical to hard rock from his collection of CDs. For all, the music is a vital part of the operating room environment, calming nerves, dissolving tension, relieving the sometimes monotonous tasks, offering moments of incredible poignancy, such as when "Tears in Heaven," Eric Clapton's popular ballad that mourns the death of his son, is cued up on the stereo. It is like anesthesia for the doctors and nurses. And the stories about the musical selections in O.R. 4 can be legendary. Fellows tell a story of Bob Goldstein becoming instantly excited during one transplant, yelling at a fellow to "Pump It Up! PUMP IT UP!" The young surgeon, frantically looking for the patient's problem, convinced suddenly that a horrible disaster was happening and he, oblivious, didn't have a clue as to how to fix it, checked blood pressure, heart rate, everything—looking for the thing he was supposed to "PUMP UP!"

"The radio—pump up the radio!" Goldstein finally declared.

The sun set outside the operating room window, and the time was near to remove Berg's liver. Van Morrison crooned about what a marvelous night it was for a moondance, and

■

43

nurses bopped about to the jazzy, romantic beat. At Berg's armpit and his groin, new cuts were made to expose major veins. The veins were opened, and large plastic tubes were fed in, then stitched to secure them in place. A third tube ran to Berg's hepatic artery, and all are connected to a machine the size of a washing machine called a "veno-veno bypass." In the early days of transplanting, once the patient was without a liver and blood circulation was curtailed, a race was on to get the new liver in and get it hooked up as quickly as possible to restore proper circulation. When the liver is out, any and all major systems in the body can fail, killing the patient. Now, the "veno-veno bypass" machine, developed by Starzl, keeps blood flowing through areas that previously were cut off, giving the surgeons a little more breathing room, a little more stability. It doesn't replace the functioning of the liver, doesn't provide the artificial support of a heart-lung bypass machine, which can oxygenate blood and provide proper pumping, or of a kidney dialysis machine, which can actually cleanse impurities from blood much the way a human kidney does. The day may come soon when an "artificial liver" moves into the operating room, but for now, the veno-veno bypass just provides a little more comfort to the surgeons.

"Ready to go on bypass."

"Bypass on."

"Turn up the music please. This is good music here," Klintmalm shouted, as Van Morrison harmonized about taking away sadness and easing troubles.

"We need to get the liver up" and out of the cooler, Klintmalm declared.

On a back table, the cooler was opened and the cellophane bag tightly shut with sneaker laces was cut open. GK reached in and lifted out the brown blob of liver, smooth and shiny and dripping wet, the odd-looking and unlikely focus of so much attention. He set it in a stainless steel bowl, like some ready-to-serve dish. Fourteen hours before, it had been in Tyler,

■

Texas, in another home, and all day it had been the subject of a life-and-death drama.

Klintmalm and Distant traded places. Berg's was a complicated plumbing job, and the day had grown past long. There would be another time to let a surgical fellow try something like this himself. But tonight was not the night.

"Bypass flow?" Klintmalm asked.

"Two liters," the answer came.

Snip, snip, cut.

"OK, liver coming out," Klintmalm said, shaking the organ out over a towel as if it were a fresh head of just-washed lettuce and then plopping it into a plastic Tupperware tub.

"Clamp," Klintmalm requested. "Another clamp. Turn down the music now."

As many times as he had done it, the tension still built. Inside Berg was an empty cavity lying before his diaphragm, which looked like a translucent cloth covering the beating heart just to the north. No longer a monument to artistic beauty, someone had taken an ax to the Matisse cutout. At this moment, Berg's belly looked hardly human, naked as a car would look without an engine or an airplane without wings.

Klintmalm, having decided it was too late and everyone was too tired to have Distant sew in this liver, donned his "loupes"—glasses fixed with special magnifying lenses for fine microsurgery.

The brown blob of liver was placed onto the surgical table just below its new home. Like its predecessor, it was shaken of dripping fluid. Then it rested on top of Berg's towel-covered groin, sitting there like a piece of meat awaiting the grill. Klintmalm began trimming vessels to approximate lengths to match Berg's plumbing, then began sewing long, tiny threads of prolene—silklike plastic—from inside the abdomen, out over the blue sterile paper and cloth covering Berg, and finally a foot or more away to the matching vessels on the donor liver. It all looked like a web of tiny telephone wires.

■

In four minutes, Klintmalm had the liver wired and lifted into Berg's abdomen, tightening the threads as he went. Speed, after all, is his trademark. He is a master tactician in the operating room, smooth, steady, and swift. In minutes, he sewed together Berg's upper vena cava to the new liver's vena cava stub, then the lower vena cava stub to Berg's insides, and then grabbed the portal vein.

Inside the liver is a maze of cells that produce vital chemicals and a myriad of ducts that carry blood through the organ. While it sits in the cooler, transplant surgeons have found, potassium and other chemicals accumulate. When blood reenters the liver, the chemicals get swept away and become a dangerous shock to the body, possibly causing heart failure. So the liver is flushed before the final hookups, with solution fed in through the portal vein above the liver.

Flush completed, Klintmalm moved into overdrive to finish the transplant. He took the portal vein and opened it wide, stretching it so that it looked like the mouth of a baby bird begging for a worm from its mother. He muttered about the condition of the vein and began sewing, working like a jewel cutter with a rock-solid left hand holding the vein and a dexterous right hand, the smooth, clever one, gliding a curved needle through the tissue. It took only the tiniest of movements to get the job done. The sewing movements were so delicate, so fine, so specific that it seemed almost like a seamstress trying to put a needle through a piece of thread, rather putting the thread through the eye of the needle.

"Unclamp in five minutes," he warned.

"Oh, shit!"

Klintmalm's exclamation drew sudden attention from the nurses, surgeons, and anesthesiologists. He had been sewing and tying at his familiar rapid pace. Now he was holding a broken thread in his hand, the needle it had been attached to instantaneously lost. Eyes turned to Berg's belly, where the lilliputian needle might be mucking around, until Klintmalm

■

found it stuck in his rubber glove. With a new glove on, he repaired the damaged suture to the portal vein and announced, "Open vena cava. Now opening portal vein."

With his right hand easing open the clamp that had sealed off the portal vein, Klintmalm stared at the machine beeping with Berg's heartbeats and measuring his pulse, blood pressure, and other vital statistics. It is the most crucial moment of the transplant, both for the surgeon and the anesthesiologist, the time when blood is returned to the new liver. Always, there is an immediate drop in blood pressure as the new liver sucks up its supply of the recipient's blood. Some unstable patients crash and die at this moment, either from an influx of chemicals from the new liver (flushed, but not completely clean) or from changes in pressure. And then there is the danger of bleeding. If there has been an injury to the liver, or if the newly sewn connections are not all leakproof, the patient can begin bleeding rapidly, sometimes fatally. Klintmalm slowly, tenuously, eased Berg's new liver back to life, even as the anesthesiologist was laughing and telling jokes.

"Well, you weren't that cocky the last time they arrested," Klintmalm chuckled, removing the clamp completely.

Blood seeped through the liver, and it turned from brown to a paisley of purple and red, with swirls and marble-like color sweeping through it as it awoke from a 14-hour slumber. It was one of those moments when man has clearly defied the gods, able to fill a cavity inside Mel Berg, where once a useless liver had rested, with a new, healthy organ that yesterday had kept alive a different father of five. It was a triumph not just of surgery but also of the human compassion and understanding that prompted the family in Tyler, Texas, to donate the organ to a stranger who will never be known to them. Life, dark red and purple life, oozed through Mel Berg's new liver, immediately putting it to work.

Klintmalm now began working on the other blood supply to the liver—the hepatic artery. Much smaller and more delicate than the vein, the artery carries almost as much flow under much higher pressure. It is also the sole source of blood for the bile duct system. GK began sewing with a needle finer than a human hair. If he skims too lightly through the wall of the artery, it can break open and the patient could bleed very seriously. If he catches the back wall of the vessel as he sews, he could unknowingly strangle it shut and choke off blood supply. One twitch could mean the difference between a successful transplant and an unsuccessful one.

Another suture broke as he tied a knot. "What is this? Holy sheeeet!" he stammered. "I'm not used to having them break. Something's wrong here."

A third broke after that, but by 9 P.M., Klintmalm had the artery open, and little if any bleeding was found inside Berg. After noting to Distant that Berg's bile duct is diseased, and the new bile duct should be routed right into the intestines, rather than into Berg's native bile duct, he stripped off his gloves and gown and headed for a break in the surgeon's lounge.

"I think it was good for you to see how we removed the portal vein thrombosis," he said to Distant, referring to the ballooning of the vein that required an extensive alternation in the usual surgery. "The first time Bo [Husberg, one of Klintmalm's surgeons] saw that, his jaw dropped."

Distant went back to work on the lead surgeon's side, cutting and burning off the gall bladder on the new liver as a mournful, yet appropriate, Neil Young song came on the stereo: "Old Man."

Tension eased, nurses chatted and began trying to predict what time they would finish. Distant worked to sew the bile duct in to the reconfigured intestines and inserted a "baby feeding tube" inside to keep the delicate duct open for the first few months after the surgery.

Sixty minutes later, Klintmalm was back, moving in to inspect the handiwork.

■

"I hate to say this, but I think there's some bleeding from down here," he said, lifting the liver up out of its cavity.

Both surgeons took argon coagulators, space-age wands that stop bleeding with a burn, and began blasting away at the underside of the liver. The bright-blue electric-like flame sealed any spots on the liver, and on Berg's inch-thick chest wall, from which he might be bleeding. As Distant finished tying Berg's bile duct, Klintmalm offered suggestions on the proper tension. Too hard, and the anastomosis—the point where the two vessels are tied together—might leak. Leave a little room for healing, but not too much room, because a too-loose tie might leak as well. He began making demonstration stitches in the muscle and tissue of Berg's open chest wall, leaving a little extra silk inside Berg while teaching. As advanced as the science of transplanting has come, success rates and patient survival sometimes come down to little tricks and special feels—how hard to tie the knots. A snag on the back wall of a bile duct may mean a trip back to the operating room, or worse, for the patient. Some have died, bile backing up and drowning the liver in its own juice. A leak may mean infection and numerous complications in the abdomen. "It's the fine points that make a difference, you know," Klintmalm said. "You can't describe the feel in bile duct stitches. What is too strong? What is not strong enough? It's like the color green—it's hard to describe, but you know it when you see it. After a while, you know the difference."

After radioactive dye was injected into the bile duct system for an X ray, which showed all was open and operating well, Klintmalm headed for the locker room to change and go upstairs to report to Berg's family while Distant sewed his abdomen closed.

It was midnight, again.

"Everything went fine. He's doing well," Klintmalm said to the family, now suddenly much larger than at 4 P.M. All four other children, and some spouses, had flown in to Dallas that night while GK was in O.R. 4 and reached Baylor from Arizona, Illinois, Colorado, and Florida to join their mother and sister at the vigil while the transplant was taking place.

They all looked tense, yet sleepy, and speechless, eyes glazed with stars as they scrutinized Klintmalm in wonder.

"How old was the donor?" one asked.

"It was a 58-year-old donor."

"How bad was his liver?" Connie Berg asked. "We thought he was doing so much better lately, that maybe it had gotten better?"

"No, it was very diseased," Klintmalm said. "He had only about six months to live."

They gasped. "Six months." The words hung very heavy.

"Thank God it all went well. Oh, thank God," they said together.

Rob, Berg's oldest son, was mesmerized by Klintmalm, as most are when the surgeons come up to the fourteenth floor with news of the miracle.

"All we can say is, thank you," he sputtered.

Then everyone shook Klintmalm's hand as he left, a god in their eyes.

"Well, my last meal was toast and orange juice eleven hours ago," Klintmalm said, once on an elevator. "I think I'll go home now."

CHAPTER 4
THE DREAM

It has always been the surgeon's dream: Take apart the body, reach over to a table for a new part, and put it in. The fantasy stretches back to Greek mythology, when a beast called The Chimera had a lion's head, a goat's body, and a dragon's fiery breath and long, scaly tail. In the second century A.D., according to a Christian story, the saints Cosmos and Damian amputated a patient's leg and replaced it with a leg from a man who had recently died. By the sixteenth century, the Italian healer Gaspare Tagliacozzi wrote a book titled *On the Surgery of Mutilation by Grafting Techniques.* The Roman Catholic church did not approve, saying the Italian was doing the devil's work by interfering with the "will of God." While historians don't doubt the veracity of the ancient surgical claims, few medical experts believe any of them were successful. Yet by the eighteenth century, when the British Empire extended to India, British surgeons discovered skin grafting techniques there that were said to date back to 300 B.C. Soon noses and corneas were grafted onto recipients.

In the early twentieth century, the dream of The Chimera began taking shape again. Alexis Carrel, first in Lyon, France, and then in Chicago, developed a technique to sew blood vessels together. He then performed the first transplants in animals, giving a dog a new heart, a cat a new kidney. The *New York Herald,* on June 2, 1906, was impressed:

CAN ALTER BLOOD CURRENTS AT WILL
Chicago Surgeons Discover
Method of Transposing
Circulatory System.

MAY TRANSPLANT ORGAN

By Changing Veins Into Arteries
Fresh Vital Fluid Can Be Sent
Into Diseased Areas

Opens New Surgical Field

Hitherto Incurable Diseases of Heart, Liver
And Brain Can Be Reached By New Method

Carrel abandoned organ transplanting, however, convinced that he could not overcome the barrier of "non-self." He didn't know what it was, but knew it was there. The laws of nature were stacked against him, and Carrel chose to explore manufacturing artificial organs, teaming with aviation pioneer Charles Lindbergh for one invention: a pulsing pump to perfuse organs, something akin to an artificial heart. In 1912, Carrel was awarded the Nobel Prize.

The field of transplanting was moving quickly, however, even without Carrel. In 1906, Frenchman Mathieu Jaboulay took a kidney from a pig and transplanted it into a dying woman. The same year he tried a goat liver in another female patient. Both died. In 1936, two Russians attempted a human kidney transplant from a cadaver. The kidney produced small amounts of urine for two days, then stopped, and the patient died on Day Four.

In the 1940s, Sir Peter Medawar produced the most important breakthrough in transplanting by identifying and describing the human immune system, the body's ability to

■

distinguish between friend and foe and fight off and kill invading viruses and bacteria. It is the immune system that allows us to vaccinate populations against disease and permits the body to heal itself in times of crisis. It is also the immune system that attacks transplanted organs. The key to transplanting, suddenly, appeared to be finding a way to suppress or trick the immune system.

Kidneys clearly were the easiest of the organs to transplant by this time, and research focused there. In 1947, the Peter Bent Brigham Hospital in Boston, Massachusetts, stepped to the forefront, with surgeon David Hume making a claim to perhaps the first successful human transplant. Hume sewed a kidney into a woman in a coma. She improved as the transplanted kidney purified her blood. When her own kidneys revived after one day, Hume removed the additional kidney. The patient woke up.

Three years later, a patient in Chicago survived six months with a transplanted kidney, grabbing worldwide media attention and exciting surgical pioneers.

The Brigham, as it's known, stepped forward in the '50s with the first real, long-term success: Joseph E. Murray, who had replaced Hume, performed a 1954 kidney transplant between a pair of identical twins. Given the same genetic makeup, the recipient's immune system classified the new kidney as familiar, friendly material and accepted it as its own. Four years later, Murray transplanted the first kidney using total body irradiation to suppress the immune system.

Still, success was fleeting, and enthusiasm for transplantation was waning. Moratoriums were considered, and scrapping the whole endeavor seemed likely. The National Academy of Sciences organized a fateful conference in September 1963 for American, French, English, and Scottish surgical pioneers, as well as immunologists including Medawar. Virtually all of the world's transplant expertise was

■

collected in one room, and there were fewer than thirty people there all together. Two hundred forty-four transplants had been performed worldwide, and failure was almost universal. Only nine survived for more than a year; six of the nine were kidneys from relatives. Only in identical twins was there any sign of success. About sixty percent of those transplants survived more than one year. Was it ethical to continue?

Then a young, self-trained transplant surgeon from Denver, Thomas E. Starzl, began presenting his results. Armed with his patient charts rolled up under his arm because he knew the audience of famous skeptics would be taken aback by what he had to say, Starzl reported that eighteen of twenty-seven successive kidney recipients over the previous ten months, all "terminal" at the time of transplant, were alive with good renal function. The results were better when the donor and recipient were related (almost eighty percent successful). No one could have dreamed of it then, but one of the patients would go on to live thirty years.

The difference? Starzl had begun using a "cocktail" of immunosuppressive drugs: azathioprine, which is an antimetabolite drug known as Imuran, along with a steroid called prednisone. Both inhibit the work of lymphocytes, the killer cells that attack foreign cells in the body. Imuran helped by destroying lymphocytes. Steroids were shown to slow down the attacking process in the liver. Even today, it is not totally understood how the steroids work in the immune system, although it is believed that they penetrate lymphocyte cellular membranes and reduce production.

"At the formal meetings, I found it difficult to speak," Starzl recalled in his memoirs, *The Puzzle People*. "It may have been my insecurity in the presence of such important dignitaries which caused me to be uneasy. In addition, I felt like someone who had parachuted unannounced from another planet onto turf that was already occupied. I was the only American transplant surgeon who had no exposure to the

■

Harvard system and experience. However, although I had never been to any other transplant center including the Brigham, I was keenly aware of what had been done by the others who had gathered for the conference."

Following the meeting, several of the participants went to Denver to see what Starzl was doing. He won them over, and soon a kidney boom was on, everyone scrambling to catch up. Starzl had created a monster. By the summer of 1964, there were 200 kidney transplant centers in the country, all trying to take the procedure to the populace, and cash in at the same time. Suddenly, the science was driven by money, and the best interests of the patients appeared secondary to ill-equipped surgeons and hospitals rushing into transplantation without proper know-how. The supply of cadaver kidneys disappeared as they were allocated quickly to the best paying customers, not the sickest patients.

Starzl, that year, was in no way resting on his achievements. He transplanted six baboon kidneys into humans but had no success. It was a pattern he would repeat thirty years later in Pittsburgh, when, in 1992, his team would transplant two baboon livers into humans. Both patients died within a short time.

Tom Starzl had begun his medical career thinking he would find a cure for cancer, only to read in 1958 that such a cure was "around the corner." In 1963, the son of a small-town Iowa newspaper editor set his laser-sharp and relentless sights on his primary prize: the liver, the organ of life whose name is derived from the verb to live. Unlike in modern culture, Shakespeare placed the liver in first position on his famous list: "Liver, brain and heart, these sovereign thrones" (*Twelfth Night*, Act 1, Scene 1). Starzl knew that the liver, which holds one-quarter of the body's blood at rest, is responsible for a myriad of vital tasks, such as manufacturing and releasing one thousand different enzymes, extracting ammonia from amino acids, absorbing fat and converting carbohydrates, manufactur-

■

ing blood proteins and coagulants, processing milk sugar (lactose) into glucose, storing some vitamins and proteins, and cleansing the body of poisons. He believed the organ held far more promise for curing disease than kidneys. And it was far more challenging. For several years in his research lab he had been attempting to transplant livers between dogs, some of whom lived for more than 100 days.

"Livers were always the jewel," said Starzl, sitting in his cluttered office and reflecting on the past, while at the same time racing to complete another research paper before a deadline. "Kidneys were just a step to that."

On March 1, 1963, Starzl attempted the world's first human liver transplant. It was a milestone little noticed at the time.

Starzl tried to cure a three-year-old boy of a fatal genetic disease by giving him a new liver. But Bennie Solis bled to death on the operating room table, reducing surgeons and nurses to tears. All four other liver-transplant recipients died that year, casting a pall over the liver program and prompting a three-year self-imposed moratorium.

Until the late 1960s, it had always been assumed that organs would come from cadavers whose hearts had stopped beating and who were declared "dead." Most of these people could not breathe for themselves and were only kept "alive" by a breathing machine called a ventilator. "Pulling the plug"— disconnecting the breathing machine—was a concept that the public accepted. For donation, the plug first had to be pulled, and then, after the heart stopped and death was pronounced, organs could be removed. By definition, any liver or kidney would have lost its blood supply inside the donor. Carving out organs from bodies whose hearts were still beating was a grim picture, and one that did not sit comfortably with all segments of society. David Hume, now in Richmond, Virginia, was once arrested and charged with murdering donors—accused of actually causing the death because the prosecutor thought the

■

donor was "alive" when the heart was still beating, even if it was only beating because of help from a machine. The case was dismissed.

In 1966, at a medical meeting in London, a new concept was introduced: the "heart-beating" cadaver. It was the first time the idea of brain death had been raised, and it would prove crucial to the success of transplantation. The public responded positively to the concept of brain death, even the Catholic church weighing in with its approval. Soon, brain death was accepted into law in the United States.

On December 3, 1967, transplantation was jolted again. Christiaan Barnard, a little-known South African who had trained in the United States and was anxious to make history, took the heart of a twenty-five-year-old woman and sewed it into a fifty-four-year-old greengrocer. "Jesus, it's going to work," Barnard was said to have exclaimed in Afrikaans. The operation of four hours and forty-five minutes was perceived as one of the great historic events of the twentieth century and transformed Barnard into an instant celebrity.

"Lurid fiction had become scientific fact and the distinctions between life and death had become blurred and rearranged," *Newsweek* magazine gushed after the Barnard feat.

There was grumbling in medical circles, of course. Several other teams were better prepared to be the first and had been beaten by Barnard. The first operation, the establishment said, should have been the honor of Norman Shumway of Stanford University, who, after all, had been the one to develop the surgical technique in dogs that would be used in human heart transplantation. But Shumway had been delayed while seeking the necessary approval from the United States Food and Drug Administration. He ended up being the second man to transplant a human heart. (He also once ended up getting arrested for "murdering" a donor, but that case, too, was dismissed.)

■

Barnard's first patient died of pneumonia eighteen days after the transplant. The next month, the surgeon tried again, four days before Shumway's first try. Denton Cooley and Michael DeBakey joined the heart transplant fray a few months later in the summer of 1968. By the end of that tumultuous year in politics and in science, a total of 102 heart transplants had been attempted worldwide; sixty percent of the patients had died.

Was Barnard a hero or a dangerous opportunist for letting the genie out of the bottle? He is not only credited with the first human heart transplant, but also with unleashing an epidemic of premature transplants. Felix Rapaport, editor of the journal *Transplantation Proceedings* and a leading American historian of transplantation, says Barnard's surgery was "one of the lowest points in transplant history." Yet Barnard's friends say he is the victim of medical jealousy. "He did the first, and it took lots of guts and courage," said Dr. Nazih Zuhdi, who trained with Barnard in Minnesota and has remained a close friend ever since. "Nobody can take that credit away from him. Nobody."

In Denver, Tom Starzl was transplanting again, spurred on by new advances and the worldwide excitement about transplants. He even began transplanting multiple organs, performing a heart-kidney transplant on September 15, 1968. The recipient died after the operation.

In the sometimes staid and conservative world of medicine, Tom Starzl, maverick, was becoming tagged with a reputation as a lunatic, perhaps even a danger. He had been taken to task at a 1965 conference for the use of convicts as kidney donors. Questions were mounting about his poor success rates. What was the point if most were dying? Shut him down, some said.

Starzl and a handful of others around the world, notably Roy Calne in England, persevered in doing liver transplants despite the number of dying patients. He developed a way to reroute blood in the patient during surgery. He developed better surgical techniques, better ways to harvest organs, better ways to preserve them outside the body, and a biopsy technique to provide early detection of rejection by hunting under a microscope for encroaching killer cells. In the process, he demonstrated the liver's role in glucose absorption for diabetics, and he showed that blood-clotting factors came from the liver.

Still, criticism mounted. Some thought Starzl ought to have his medical license revoked, and there were even rumors of a movement in Denver medical circles to shut him down, though Starzl says he never heard such gossip. Others recognized him as a genius. He was at war with the medical establishment, too, over the explosion of kidney transplanting centers in the '70s. Starzl detested the spread of kidney transplanters, saying it was a national scandal that kidneys were being allocated only to the rich. A bureaucracy created to control the situation simply made for a second problem. He also argued that it was unethical to take kidneys from living relatives, since a small percentage of donors—otherwise perfectly healthy people trying to help a family member—die, violating the physicians' credo to "First, do no harm." It is a conviction he still maintains today; his transplant service doesn't perform such living-relative transplants.

Starzl exited the kidney business in 1972 to concentrate totally on livers. By the end of the 1970s, he had by far the best success rate in the world, but still just thirty of one hundred liver cases survived for more than one year. DeBakey and others had given up on transplanting hearts. Too many patients died. To most, it was not worth the battle. Transplanting began to look like a dead dream, a massive failure—to just about everyone but Tom Starzl.

Why did he continue in the face of such adversity, he was asked in an interview.

"There has to be a conviction," he said simply.

And why did he continue when others were calling him a lunatic who was killing patients?

"I guess I didn't hear them," he said with a sly smile.

In 1970, a miraculous discovery was made. Sandoz Pharmaceuticals, a Swiss drug company, routinely asked its employees to bring back soil samples from foreign vacations to test for new substances that might produce new drugs. That year, some soil came from Norway containing a previously unknown fungus, named *Tolypocladium inflatum*, which was cultured in hopes it might produce a new antibiotic. The fungus produced a substance labeled cyclosporine for its cyclical polypeptides, and it was investigated because it revealed in test tubes to have some antifungal properties—it might be able to kill some fungus infections.

The new director of the department doing the investigation at Sandoz, Jean Borel, observed something else about this cyclosporine: It was able to inhibit lymphocyte cultures without destroying the surrounding cells. Lymphocytes—the cells of the immune system that attack foreign cells—had been the thorny problem of transplantation. The body needs them to fight off disease, so getting rid of them totally is out of the question. But they attack the transplanted organs as unfriendly invaders. What was remarkable about cyclosporine was that it appeared to inhibit only part of the immune apparatus, a subgroup of lymphocytes called T-cells. If cyclosporine could target these killer cells, without destroying the entire immune system, it might be just the discovery transplanters were waiting for. The first paper on this new development was published in 1976.

A sample was sent to Roy Calne in Cambridge, England, and he found it was far superior to anything else used as an immunosuppressor. But there was also a problem: Cyclosporine damaged the kidneys it was supposed to protect. In 1979, Calne reported side effects to cyclosporine, including

■

severe nephrotoxicity and high incidence of lymphomas—cancers of the immune system. What's more, Borel had to fight Sandoz executives fiercely to convince them there was a market for the drug big enough to justify the manufacturing cost. The program was killed at one point, and Calne and a young immunologist at Cambridge, David White, flew to Basel, Switzerland, to successfully appeal the corporate decision. Still, with the kidney and cancer problems, cyclosporine was looking more and more like a dead dream.

Meanwhile, Starzl, still in Denver and working now with a new fellow, Goran Klintmalm of Sweden, tried giving the new drug in combination with steroids and Imuran, as a kind of "cocktail." The doses of cyclosporine required were much lower when used with steroids, with the side effects greatly reduced. Starzl's results on "triple drug therapy," published with Klintmalm listed as the second author, saved the drug and paved the way for another transplant goldrush.

Cyclosporine was approved by the Food and Drug Administration in 1980 for experimental treatment, and then fully approved in 1983. One-year survival rates soared for transplanting, with the liver success rate climbing from thirty percent for one-year survival to more than sixty percent.

But Starzl's Denver program wouldn't survive. The program began unraveling when two key players in the transplantation staff were fired, and it became clear that the hospital administration was withdrawing its support of its controversial risk taker. Searching for a new home, Starzl and surgeon Shun Iwatsuki thought about Los Angeles but decided on Pittsburgh, where he and his program, including fellows Goran Klintmalm and Carlos Fernandez-Bueno of Puerto Rico, were taken in by Henry T. Bahnson, Starzl's best man at his first wedding and the chairman of the Department of Surgery at Presbyterian University Hospital.

By 1983, liver transplanting was approved by the United States government as an accepted medical treatment for a variety of diseases. Insurance companies began paying for the surgery, and the boom was on. There would be no turning back this time.

The number of patients banging on the door quickly outstripped the capacity. Only a handful of people in the world had the training and talent to undertake this new art of liver transplanting, and Starzl-trained fellows quickly became hot commodities.

Soon an old friend called Starzl from Dallas. It was John Fordtran, one of the foremost experts on diseases of the digestive tract, inquiring about help in setting up a transplant program at Baylor University Medical Center. No one else in that part of the country was venturing into livers—not even Houston, which had become the mecca for hearts.

Fordtran and Starzl had a special bond. Fordtran, a distinguished internist, had gone to Denver in 1971 not as a physician but as the father of a patient. Billy Fordtran, like two of his three siblings, had an inherited disease fatal to kidneys. It was discovered in 1965, when Billy was nine, and by 1971, he was in kidney failure.

"At the time, it was like a death sentence," Fordtran recalled. "Even dialysis was not available, and transplants had really only been successfully done in identical twins.

"People started mentioning the name Starzl to us. It was a name I had never heard before, but it was like a breath of fresh air. He assumed everything was going to be OK. He had a positive attitude and was ready to fight. He was so confident and reassuring, he gave us hope. Then, when we went to see him, we were taken aback at how young he looked."

The Fordtrans showed up in that dark period in transplanting when Starzl was at war with the kidney establishment and embattled over the lack of success in livers. He planned to transplant a kidney from Fordtran's wife, Jewel, to her son. But on the afternoon of the scheduled surgery, a cadaver kidney became available in Denver. Even though the results for cadaver transplants in 1971 were far worse than transplants from relatives, the Fordtrans took Starzl's advice and chose the cadaver, primarily because three of the four children faced the same fate.

Billy did not recover well. He suffered several bouts of rejection, and remained weak. He came down with what appeared to be fatal pneumonia. Fordtran spent four months in Denver at the side of his son, and Tom Starzl. "He and I were always confiding in each other. We became very, very close friends," Fordtran said. Finally, Billy Fordtran developed a tolerance to his new kidney, recovering to finish school, become a pharmacist, marry and have a family.

In 1984, Fordtran called his old friend with a proposition. Would Starzl consider coming to Baylor? The transplant pioneer had remarried, to a medical technician from the Dallas area (Fordtran was the best man at Starzl's second wedding), so moving to Dallas would offer the chance to be close to her family. His welcome in Pittsburgh was still a bit tentative and controversial, because no one was sure if his program would bring success or scorn to the University of Pittsburgh and its hospital. Baylor offered a private, well-endowed hospital with a new facility providing plenty of beds and brand-new, empty operating rooms.

"For maybe a month or two he said he had some interest in it," Fordtran said. "And for a few months we worked on the assumption that we might be able to get him. But things developed well in Pittsburgh, and as I look back, I think a lot of it had to do with the fact that he wanted to do something for me."

Deciding to remain in Pittsburgh, Starzl offered a consolation prize. He would make the Baylor program a satellite operation to Pittsburgh. He would pick the surgeon and give him a faculty appointment at Pittsburgh as well. He would make it work for Dallas.

"There were only two people in the world with the technical skills and the administrative abilities to do it," Starzl said. "One went to Harvard, and the other was Goran."

Klintmalm remembers the phone ringing at about 11 P.M. in Stockholm one night. "As always, Tom never introduced himself. He just said, 'Hi Goran. Have you heard about Baylor?'

"I said I had heard the name.

"'Are you interested?'"

Klintmalm, who was running the cyclosporine trials in Scandinavia, came in March to visit and was impressed. He wanted a home with a research focus, not just a factory that would replace worn-out livers. Baylor was willing to commit the resources. He agreed to a deal on a handshake but insisted that Baylor had to secure for him an immigrant's visa, not just a common visa sponsored by the institution. That way, Baylor wouldn't be able to cancel his visa and force him back to Sweden.

"It took months and months to get," Klintmalm said. The program was scheduled to start the following spring.

Starzl, never one to tolerate delays and waiting, suddenly threw a wrench into the methodical preparations at Christmas.

Amie Garrison, a five-year-old girl from Texas, was dying of liver failure, and her plight had captured the attention of Nancy Reagan, whose physician-father had been one of Starzl's mentors. She held a "status four" in the organ bank computer—the most critical, likely to die soon without a transplant. A liver became available in Hamilton, Canada, on December 21, and Starzl called Baylor, saying he did not have enough accommodations for the girl in Pittsburgh. Klintmalm had not yet had time to even receive a Texas medical license. But Starzl's plan was to come to Dallas himself and do the transplant, bringing his own anesthesiologist, his own instruments, everything.

Boone Powell, Jr., president of the hospital, came back to his office late in the day to deliver Christmas gifts to his staff. Sitting there waiting for him were all the heads of Baylor's departments—the entire power structure of the hospital.

■

"What in the world has happened?" Powell asked.

Starzl was pushing, and Powell was immediately under the gun. The biggest fear at Baylor was that the program would get off to a bad start. There would be a lot of attention. Could they survive if the first patient died? What if the first five died? Now, here was Starzl, with the national media and the First Lady in tow, ready to stage a dramatic first act in the Baylor production, ready to try to save Amie Garrison and give birth to his new transplant baby in one fell swoop.

"I had not received any inappropriate advice from him at all," Powell said of Starzl. "We had a checklist and went around the room to each department. Everyone said, 'Yeah, we think we can do it.' So we activated the program."

Starzl was testing the Baylor resolve. Fordtran recognized the pattern. "I told everyone, 'I know Tom. If we don't back him up, he'll lose confidence in this institution,'" Fordtran said.

Powell called Starzl to say yes. "At the end of the conversation, he said, 'There's been some publicity about this young lady. Mrs. Reagan is involved.'

"I said I knew. Then he said, 'There's a little risk involved here, but I love it!'"

Amie Garrison survived her transplant, recovered, and continues to do extremely well. She is now a teenager.

In 1990, for the first time ever, a Nobel Prize was awarded in medicine for transplantation. The winners: Joe Murray and a Seattle researcher who came up with a breakthrough in bone-marrow transplantation. Tom Starzl, the pioneer scorned and vilified only to be proven right, was passed over. Too controversial, probably.

"It was an absolute crime when he was not included when they gave the Nobel Prize for transplantation," Fordtran said. "A lot of it was jealousy. Those people are just different from him. He's a doer, and they're not doers. I don't see how anybody could deny the enormous positive impact he's had."

To John Fordtran, it was a slight that not only offended him as a physician but also as the father of a child saved from certain death. His two daughters, stricken with the same kidney disease, went on to have transplants themselves, the beneficiary of a single unrelated donor who happened to be a nearly perfect match. His life, his family, have been changed by transplantation. There can be no greater gift than getting a child back from the dead.

"Tom Starzl made a difference, a major difference. He was the one out there saying, 'This will work.' And that makes a difference to people with sick children. It's really difficult to accept children dying. And Tom Starzl made the difference between living with hope versus living with no hope."

■

CHAPTER 5
THE DONOR COWBOYS

Caren Eisenstein slumped into the wide, slippery, leather backseat of the Lear jet and cooed: "We're the donor cowboys! Here we go again."

It was the second time this Saturday that Eisenstein had buried herself under blankets in the back of a Lear, the second time the young surgeon, a Kansas City native who had visited Pittsburgh, UCLA, and the Mayo Clinic during her transplant training and was now on a two-year transplant fellowship with Goran Klintmalm, had taxied to the end of runway 13 Right at Dallas Love Field. It was the second time she had flown to El Paso International Airport in one day.

For two weeks, there had been hardly any donors, two weeks during which Klintmalm's surgeons groused, fretted, and agonized over the declining condition of some patients waiting for organs. But now the Baylor team found itself in the middle of a marathon stretch of harvests and transplants—three livers in thirty-six hours. Klintmalm and Eisenstein had retrieved a liver from Dallas's Parkland Hospital overnight, and now that organ was being transplanted into a patient by another Swedish surgeon on Klintmalm's team, Bo Husberg.

At 10 A.M., the Southwest Organ Bank had called Klintmalm, just getting into his riding clothes for a day of polo at an exclusive Dallas club populated with business tycoons, with word of the first El Paso liver. He reached Eisenstein at her (less-exclusive) riding stable, and she had rushed to Love Field in her jodhpurs. She and Klintmalm, along with a heart transplant team from Dallas and organ bank coordinator Cindy Morphew, flew 700 miles to the Texas-Mexico border city to harvest the liver of a thirty-two-year-old soldier who, while drunk, had wandered into the street and was struck by a car. He was declared brain dead at El Paso's military hospital, and after the military organ transplant program in San Antonio, Texas, turned down an offer of his blood group O liver (the most common), the Baylor team was summoned.

Before the plane had even left the ground, that liver oozed controversy. Klintmalm had selected Jackie Henning, a thirty-four-year-old father of three near the top of the list who had been waiting four months. Henning, unemployed because of his debilitating genetic disease, had been beeped at his son's soccer game and was on his way to Baylor as Klintmalm headed for Love Field. Reached on his car phone, then Klintmalm was reminded by doctors back at Baylor that Don Bryan, the man passed over as backup for the liver that went to Yolanda Contreras, was much sicker and also a good match for the El Paso liver. Could it go to Don Bryan instead? Klintmalm chose Bryan, and Henning was called and told there had been a mistake, someone more seriously ill needed the liver.

As the Lear took off, Klintmalm's beeper went off again. The pilot placed a call to Baylor, where the revered and powerful head of the gastroenterology department, Dr. Daniel Polter, was insisting that the liver go to a seriously ill patient in the intensive care unit. The man was a sixty-one-year-old alcoholic who had already sparked intense rancor in the hospital hallways. Klintmalm's surgeons, and the social worker assigned to the transplant program, didn't believe the patient had proved any sobriety, let alone the six months required for acceptance into the transplant program. On the other hand, the team of

■

gastroenterologists argued they had a critically ill patient who would surely die soon without a new liver. The man had come before Baylor's weekly selection committee meeting at a time when the session was dominated by gastroenterologists. Klintmalm and two of his three other staff surgeons were out of town or operating, and the vote quickly went in the man's favor. After the meeting, the patient was moved to Baylor's intensive care unit, allowing him to take precedence over all other patients on the waiting list.

"I guarantee you he will be noncompliant [drinking again]," fumed one of the team's social workers, after the committee meeting. "If Klintmalm and Goldstein had been there, there's no way he would have been accepted."

Klintmalm took the message from the pilot and shrugged. "OK." Don Bryan got passed over once again—a grim game of musical livers.

The daylight flight was greeted in El Paso with word of a second donor, possibly later that afternoon. A young woman, twenty-one or so, had been at a party at four A.M. and was playing "with one of those unloaded guns"—the words of the organ bank coordinator who greeted the surgeons in El Paso. The gun had gone off, destroying the woman's brain. But there would not be time to wait and take two livers back at once, Klintmalm decided. He had the first liver out in less than two hours and by five P.M. was back in Dallas driving to Baylor with the liver, chilled on ice and preservation solution in a Coleman cooler, riding in the trunk of his BMW. He would transplant this one into the sixty-one-year-old alcoholic himself that night.

The second liver turned out to be type O as well, but it was very small, and Klintmalm thought it would be a better match for a woman in Tyler, Texas, who was on the list. Pam Fertig placed the call to her, but for the first time in years, a patient said no and turned down the liver, saying she just was not yet ready.

"Call in Don Bryan," Klintmalm told Fertig and dispatched surgeon Marlon Levy and surgical fellow Eisenstein back to El Paso for the second liver at eleven P.M.

The cycle of donating organs has a rhythm all its own. For whatever reason, most harvests come in the middle of the night. The victim is declared brain dead toward the end of the working day. The family is approached, although often relatives understanding the situation will voluntarily ask about organ donation. Once consent is obtained, care of the donor is transferred to the local organ bank, in this case the Southwest Organ Bank in Dallas. The organ bank takes steps to preserve the dead person by keeping the heart stable and pumping the body full of fluids to keep organs as ripe as possible. It's a tricky tightrope walk between life and death. Often while trying to save a victim of head trauma, doctors try to dry the patient out as much as possible—just the opposite of what the organ bank would desire. Sometimes drugs are considered which might have a slim chance of success but could irreparably harm the organs for donation. And while there is supposed to be a Chinese Wall between those medical professionals interested in organ donation and those interested in saving the near-dead patient, stories abound of transplant surgeons prowling the emergency room when trauma cases come in, even of families of those waiting for transplants seeking out families of shooting victims, or car accident victims, or "brain-bleed" victims, and saying something about "being so sorry about your sorrow and your loss, but, see, our father is upstairs about to die unless he receives a new heart, and, well, if someone has to die maybe someone can live and, maybe you could consider donating. . . ." Such anecdotes, repeated by organ bank coordinators and nurses, are more than just harmful urban myths. The tales are told with deep concern, because there may be some truth.

The organ bank has several hours of tests to run, checking for everything from the AIDS virus to hepatitis to drug use.

■

If the donor passes medically, the organ is offered to a transplant program.

In this life cycle, the calls often come around midnight, and entail a late-night/early-morning Lear jet flight to a small town. Sometimes the plane is met by a hospital employee in a van, sometimes by an ambulance, sometimes by a taxi cab, sometimes even by a limo. The harvest team goes in through the emergency room, carrying coolers and tote bags of instruments. Usually there is a team for the heart, a team for the liver, and a local surgeon for the kidneys. Sometimes the lungs are harvested, sometimes the pancreas. The more organs, the more complicated and time-consuming the harvest. Then, one by one, the teams depart back to their respective cities, landing usually before dawn. To some, it can feel like the *Invasion of the Body Snatchers*. A small flight line of jets at an airport somewhere is about to depart with the parts of a human being. They sneak in under cover of darkness, while most are sleeping, and they depart before dawn. Few know the drama that has gone on overnight; few know the tragedy someone has suffered, the gift that a family has made, and the excitement of perhaps half a dozen families scattered around the United States who will wake up that morning to a new beginning.

For Caren Eisenstein, a stylish, trendy Missourian who has become part of a very small elite of female transplant surgeons, donor surgery was as close as she was going to get to operating on humans for the current six months of her two-year fellowship with Klintmalm. She was then immersed in a research project in Baylor's animal laboratory, operating on pigs to study blood flow through the liver and how it is affected by different drugs and different steps in the transplant process. The Baylor team held out high hopes for the pig liver project, hopes that someday soon, they would be transplanting pig livers into humans. The next year, Eisenstein would be Klintmalm's senior fellow.

■

To spice up the all-night drudgery of the donor runs, Eisenstein had launched a contest among the four fellows: Who could bring back the tackiest souvenirs from the trips? In the fellows' windowless office, a shelf right above the *Sports Illustrated* swim suit calendar sent by Klintmalm, who got it as a gift from a patient, was allocated for storage of the bounty. And Eisenstein was set to win her own contest. One night, racing through Ardmore, Oklahoma, in an ambulance with Klintmalm, Eisenstein spotted a grungy bar called the "Pink Moose Saloon."

"Could we stop? Could we get something there for the contest?" she pleaded like a child asking permission to do something wrong, just once.

Klintmalm ordered the ambulance stopped. Eisenstein, dressed in green surgical scrubs, raced in with an organ-bank coordinator. They bought T-shirts, bumper stickers, and even a silly plastic pink moose from the saloon, then jumped back in the ambulance to resume the task of saving a life. Back in Dallas, the plunder was proudly displayed in the office, the benchmark for all to beat.

"GK loved it. It was really fun," Eisenstein said of the Pink Moose foray.

Too tired for worrying about loot on this run, Caren Eisenstein was asleep when the Lear touched down a second time in El Paso, this time at 12:15 A.M., now Sunday. The same ambulance driver greeted the surgeons with a chuckle. "Haven't I seen you before today?"

"I think it was actually yesterday," she said, yawning.

"This city is going crazy this weekend," the driver offered. "The hospitals are jammed. Only one emergency room was still open last night here. They're all crawling with people, waiting, and the trauma areas are clogged."

R.E. Thomason General Hospital was indeed crawling with people, some lined up in the driveway to the emergency room, all watching with curiosity as doctors in hospital scrubs jumped out of the back of an ambulance, carrying a bright orange flight bag and a couple of red-and-white beer coolers. Inside, in the middle of a large, brightly lit operating room with beige, simulated wood grain linoleum walls, lay a twenty-one-year-old Hispanic female, Margarita Zapata, the woman said to have been partying with the "unloaded" gun. She spoke only Spanish, lived in the barrio of El Paso in an apartment, attended trade school and, at the time of her death, was trying to make a better life for herself. People at the party said it was a self-inflicted gunshot wound. An accident.

Actually, the team was told, the medical examiner found no powder burns on her hands—so she had been murdered. Was it for passion? For money? Or was she just in the wrong place at the wrong time?

Everyone looked at the large wound by her right temple, halfway between the ear and the eyebrow, and the exit wound on the left side of her head. The only certainty was that earlier tonight, she indeed had been in the wrong place at the wrong time.

The Southwest Organ Bank had been unable to place the pancreas or lungs. There is less demand for those organs because successful transplantation is still extremely delicate and largely unsatisfactory. The Baylor team was asked to take out the kidneys and leave them for local transplant surgeons in El Paso. Another team from Oklahoma City arrived to take the heart.

According to gossip in hospital hallways, you can tell what organ transplant surgeons specialize in just by listening to them for a few seconds. It's all in good fun, but like most stereotyping, there is a ring of truth in the characterizations. To the heart transplant surgeon, all other organs are "lesser" organs. Nothing could be more dramatic than taking a heart out of one human, watching it go soft and become a mass of deflated muscle, then hooking it back up in the empty chest of a patient and starting it again. Heart transplanters have only

73

four hours of "ischemic time"—time when the organ can remain without blood flow outside a body—so the harvest and transplant must be carefully timed, and not a minute can be wasted.

On this night, the Oklahoma City team had about six members, nurses, residents, the lead surgeon. . . . They paraded in as if accompanied by a marching band. The doors swung open: "WE'RE HERE TO TAKE THE HEART!"

Liver surgeons often seem a bit defensive about heart surgeons, some of whom they regard as pompous, self-important and inferior surgically, yet who seem to garner more attention, glory, and respect from the public. A liver transplant is the most rigorous, difficult surgery there is, requiring lilliputian work *underneath* the organ, as well as a complicated balancing act of all the body's systems. Taking out a heart or a kidney is pretty simple surgically, a cut here, a snip there. Putting in a heart is a breeze too, but it carries so much emotional baggage it comes with media attention and prominence in the medical community. Putting in a kidney is also relatively easy, too, requiring only two or three hours in the operating room. But taking out and putting in a liver are skills that only a select group of surgeons have mastered.

What's more, so many heart transplant programs have cropped up, given birth by hospitals eager for the prestige, publicity, and full beds, that few have enough work to support full-time transplant practices. In Dallas, for example, there are four heart transplant programs. To some cardiac surgeons, especially dedicated, full-time transplanters, the plethora of heart programs is a waste of medical and financial resources and a danger to patients who may not receive as much expertise as they might need.

While Margarita Zapata was dead on the table, her skin was still full of life, her heart still beating, her liver still functioning, her kidneys still producing urine. Marlon Levy watched as she was covered with blue towels and prepped for

■

surgery. As he always does, he went to her chart to check for a death certificate himself. Inside, signed consent forms for organ donation were written in Spanish. And a thank-you note for her family from the Southwest Organ Bank had already been placed in there to accompany the body to the funeral home. An anesthesiologist, working out of a red Craftsman tool drawer from Sears, placed monitors on Margarita's body and inserted tubes and needles to keep her stable through the surgery. The beeping began inside O.R. 7. Marlon Levy stepped to the front of the stage.

"Do you have some way to keep me from humming?" he asked as he prepared to begin cutting. "Is there a radio?" Anything to cover up the beep, beep, beep and to cauterize the environment.

At thirty-four, Levy is the youngest and newest of Klintmalm's trio. Born in France, he moved to Texas with his parents when he was ten at the behest of an uncle who, having been an Allied pilot in World War II during the Nazi occupation of France, had landed a job flying for American Airlines. His father worked at Neiman Marcus and raised five children in suburban Dallas. Marlon stayed in Dallas for college and medical school, trained in Wisconsin and in London, and was hired as a fellow by Klintmalm. Halfway through his fellowship, he was asked to take a staff position, doubling his fellow's salary of $30,000 or so, but not enough to replace his aging Plymouth Volare, now a thirteen-year-old paisley of pale yellow and rust.

Levy stumps through the hallways like a fast-moving, svelte Winnie the Pooh, just as his Volare kind of stumps along through traffic. He is a favorite of the patients for his relaxed, cheerful, almost happy-go-lucky mood, but he can be stern and strict when the time comes to be firm. He cuts neither the figure of the dashing surgeon nor of the brilliant researcher, but he has quickly proved himself to be both, while still looking like the kid with the stubby fingers who used to collect frogs. Once, in the pathology lab, the team examined a liver biopsy slide

■

that was diagnosed as so diseased it looked like the surface of the moon. "To the moon, Alice!" Marlon declared, doing his best Jackie Gleason, for whom he could pass as a nephew or second cousin. Another Friday afternoon, Levy noted that it was forecast to be a hot, long holiday weekend—the kind that end up busy for transplant surgeons. "There's somebody out there with my name on them, and they don't even know it," he howled.

Now, he was all business.

"Is she paralyzed?" Levy asked the anesthesiologist.

"No, sir."

"Could you please paralyze her?"

"Yes, sir."

Eighteen people have gathered in the operating room to watch as Levy began making an incision down the length of Margarita Zapata's chest, exposing her heart and her belly. Smoke rose from the body as the Bovie buzzed away, releasing the stench of burning flesh that hangs in the air like a grim reminder of just what the task at hand is. As Levy cut and the others watched, one had to wonder if so many people had ever paid this much attention to this woman before in her life.

"Can I have the saw?"

A nurse handed Levy a contraption that looked like a Black & Decker jigsaw to cut the sternum and open the chest. It was 1:10 A.M., even though the clock on the wall, still running, said 9:30. And the radio was finally on. *Walking in Memphis . . ."*

Each time the body snatchers invade a town it can seem like a clash of medical cultures. The big-time, often famous, surgeons stroll into some rinky-dink community hospital and are teamed with nurses more accustomed to C-sections and gall-bladder removals. There can be tension as commands are barked. At home, in elaborately equipped operating rooms more familiar to them than their favorite easy chair, instruments are called for by simple hand signals and nurses are

■

trained to know exactly what comes next. It can be a smooth, handcrafted eight-cylinder sports car engine pumping along. But in unfamiliar outposts in the middle of the night, the interplay between the scrub nurses and the surgeons can seem like some old jalopy hitting on only two or three cylinders. Each time, the Dallas team as a matter of course tries to crack a joke, express gratitude, and put the scrub nurses at ease early on.

The heart team moved in at the top of the chest, beginning their own dissection. One nurse near the patient's feet fed instruments to two separate operating teams, each made up of two surgeons.

A surgical resident from Oklahoma City asked for an instrument, then tossed it back at the nurse with a terse "Do you have something less gigantic?" Marlon looked at Caren, and both rolled their eyes.

Within ten minutes, the surgeons had opened the body up, transforming Margarita from somebody's daughter, somebody's sister, to a parts warehouse.

A phone stretched from the wall to the table, where one of the Oklahoma City surgeons began briefing a surgeon back home. "It's not a bad heart. The aorta is small. I think it will work. Get Mr. Crowley ready . . ."

"Our guy is very sick—but much bigger than her. He's six feet. It's very borderline, but we're going to do it," he explained to the audience.

Don Bryan, too, is over six feet tall—six feet two, in fact. He had shrunk to only 130 pounds but still about twenty pounds more than the donor. But a liver can grow to meet demand; a heart can't. The six-feet-tall Mr. Crowley will have to live with a heart not capable of keeping up with an active, large man. However, the fact is that living that way is better than dying.

"It's a beautiful liver, just beautiful," Marlon Levy was murmuring. "It's a nice crimson color with no yellow to it that would make us worry about fat."

A healthy liver is smooth and supple, with a perfectly curved leading edge so finely crafted it looks as if it came off a stealth bomber. The liver is aerodynamic, floppy yet tough, perfectly molded to fit its home inside the body. Nature does beautiful work, better than man ever will.

"Look good?" shouted Cindy Morphew, the coordinator from the organ bank who had flown out in the morning with Klintmalm and stayed all day and night in El Paso to work both donors. If the liver didn't look good, more tests might be necessary, more plans might have to be changed.

"Major-league good," Eisenstein replied.

Levy pawed aside handfuls of intestines and began feeling down under the liver for the hepatic artery—the main blood supply to the liver. Unlike the tidy pictures in textbooks, the human anatomy can be a confusing jumble of like-looking parts. Many people have abnormal anatomies—bodies that work just fine but don't have textbook-perfect structures. Without the tags and markers of multicolored pictures, Levy and Eisenstein began the tricky process of identifying and separating the hepatic artery from the splenic artery and the gastric artery and the branches of other arteries. Some vessels are no wider than the head of a pencil. Some are embedded in tissue, hidden by nature without any regard for the future possibility of organ transplantation. Since arteries pulse with each heartbeat, however, they often can be found by knowing how and where to feel.

Once found, the artery was isolated and prepared for the dissection. With control of the hepatic artery, the surgeons would be able to salvage the liver should the patient crash—and donors are by definition unstable since the body begins deteriorating as soon as the brain dies, no matter how skilled the preservation is. Systematically, Levy and Eisenstein exclude every organ not wanted, and isolate and preserve blood flow only to the ones to be transplanted—the liver and two kidneys.

■

Suddenly the donor's blood pressure dropped, and one of the "heart boys" asked if the anesthesiologist could give her some blood. It seemed rather strange, giving blood to a dead woman. What a struggle it is to keep a dead woman "alive."

The radio belted out sad love songs about heartache and pain. After thirty minutes or so, the heart team was prepared and headed to the doctors' lounge while waiting for the liver team to finish its preparations. Both organs must be taken out at the same moment.

Tension had built between the two teams. A heart surgeon standing behind Levy barked to a nurse, "Maybe you could ask the liver team to wet a cloth from time to time with warm saline and place it over the heart?"

Eisenstein asked for a bigger "right angle," a surgical instrument.

"A 'more gigantic' one," Levy crowed. "As opposed to 'less gigantic.'" The instrument nurse chuckled.

Levy and Eisenstein tied off the arteries they didn't need and controlled the aorta above and below the liver. There are five connections to be made in a liver transplant: the hepatic artery, the vena cava above and below the liver, the portal vein, and the bile duct. Everything else is discarded.

"Now we're going after the common bile duct," Levy announced, raising his voice to a crescendo.

"Kids, don't try this at HOME!"

With fine silk thread, the duct was tied twice, then cut between the two knots. The end of the sealed duct attached to the liver then will be sewn together with the recipient's bile duct during the transplant.

After the bile duct, Eisenstein worked to find the portal vein, separating it from the tissue in which it is imbedded with tiny, tiny twitches from the opening and closing of a right angle instrument. Bit by tiny bit, the vein pulled away from its nest.

"I mean, is that beautiful or what?" Levy asked

Eisenstein as he taught her technique. "See how that opened everything up?"

Eisenstein began threading a large, clear plastic tube into the portal vein, tying around it to secure it. Fluid, chilled almost to ice, was fed into the tube.

"Please start the pre-cool," she said.

At 2:40 A.M., Levy asked a nurse to tell the heart surgeons, "We're ready to go."

But Oklahoma City was not ready to go, not yet far enough along in the preparation of the recipient to allow the team in El Paso to remove the heart and start the four-hour clock running.

The heart team began stalling. "Can you show me the heart, please?" one asked, requesting that a wet cloth covering the heart be lifted. "The heart looks a little over fluid, bulging perhaps. Can we do something about that?"

Levy, in no mood at this hour on this weekend to wait with this heart team, suggested that the heart looked just fine. The other heart surgeon, the resident with the penchant for "less gigantic" instruments, asked if he could take out lymph nodes for testing before the heart was removed.

Eyes rolled again.

The heart team scrubbed their arms and hands again for sterile conditions, as everyone else stood waiting. The heart, exposed to the linoleum walls, kept beating. It looked futile, as if it never got the message that Margarita was dead. And thankfully, it never did get the message. For the heart and the liver and the two kidneys, it wasn't over yet. They would find new homes, changing the lives of four different people.

"You know, we did see some trauma in the chest," one of the heart surgeons said, chitchatting. "Who reports that to the coroner?"

No one responded.

Now the heart team wanted to inject more medication to see how the heart would respond. Fourteen people watched as the lead heart surgeon tinkered with his toy. Finally, he prepared to cut out the heart.

"Ready to slow flush. Slow. Slow. Slower now. Slower. Stop now. What is the time?"

3 A.M.

The aorta was clamped, and now the body was flooded with icy slush to rapidly cool the organs and preserve them. Fluid flowed into the heart and liver through tubes, and pitchers of slush were dumped into the body, turning the abdomen into a soup kettle of intestines and organs, a loose, bloody stew.

"*Oh, mercy, mercy me.*

"*Things ain't what they used to be . . .*" Robert Palmer sang on the radio.

With a few more snips, the heart was lifted out, rushed to a table in the back of the room, cleaned up a bit and dropped into a bag of chilly preservation solution. The bag was tied, then placed in another fluid-filled bag and sealed. It floated in the middle of the bag as if suspended inside an aquarium.

At 3:25 A.M., Caren Eisenstein lifted out the liver, smooth as an eel and now pale brown without blood, almost a stone color, or slate gray. The liver was hooked to a clear plastic tube stretching to an IV pole, still receiving an infusion of preservation fluid. It—the liver—was the patient now, followed everywhere by its bag of fluid and pole-on-wheels. Like the heart, it was cleaned up, double bagged and placed in the cooler, along with glass jars of extra lengths of arteries for patching, lymph nodes, and a piece of spleen for laboratory testing. By 4 A.M., the thank-yous were said to the nurses and the ambulance, sirens ablaze for no reason other than tradition and the thrill of the young ambulance driver, returned once again to El Paso International.

"Do you ever forget where you are on nights like this?" Marlon Levy was quizzed.

"I never ask," he responded. "I know wherever I am, I'm not going to be there very long."

■

81

Pumped up, Levy scurried onto the plane, flopped down in the rear seat that stretched the width of the jet, and spread out.

"Have you ever gone vertical?" he asked innocently. "Mike's the pilot, and Mike loves to go vertical."

Mike aimed the Lear jet, an achievement of power that itself can defy the laws of nature by rocketing through the air on tiny wings and huge engines, toward the east, back to Dallas. To the west of the El Paso airport are mountains, to the south Mexico, to the north the White Sands Missile Range. But to the east, there is nothing but desert.

"Lifeguard Eighty-three Echo-Alpha, cleared for takeoff."

At 150 miles per hour, Mike lifted the Lear off the ground, maybe 500 feet or so above the desert floor, and leveled off.

"Here he goes," Marlon cried.

If there is one distinguishing characteristic of transplant surgeons it is that they all, deep down, are thrill-seekers. There are far easier ways to make tons of money in medicine, far simpler ways to perform life-saving feats. It is a young person's profession, a profession that requires enough ego to have the confidence to defy the gods and remake a person. More than anything, though, to endure the twenty-four-hour days, the four A.M. flights, the tension of taking apart a human body and putting it back together, you have to be a thrill-seeker.

"Here he goes!"

Mike accelerated the Lear, keeping it just off the ground at the same low altitude, close enough to see moonlit cactus race by faster and faster as the jet built momentum. Two hundred miles per hour. More. Much more. Like an F-16 evading radar by ducking under the horizon, Mike hugged the desert floor, the Lear going faster and faster and faster, the liver stowed behind Levy's seat.

"HERE HE GOES!!!!!"

■

In an instant, in the time that it took to pull the trigger that ended Margarita Zapata's life, Mike pulled the Lear straight up. Vertical. There is not a roller coaster on Earth that could duplicate the speed or the sensation of leaving your stomach on the floor of the desert while you climb ten thousand feet in seconds.

Levy screamed in the back, his legs dancing and pumping at the thrill.

"YEEEEEEEEEEEE HAAAAAAAAAAA."

The donor cowboys were heading home.

At Love Field, the day not yet ready for the sun, Caren Eisenstein plopped the cooler in the trunk of her Hyundai and, without any of the sirens that had brought the liver to the airplane in El Paso, drove toward Baylor at about 5:30 A.M., nearly eighteen hours and twenty-eight hundred miles after she was summoned from the riding stable. Her rock group bumper sticker over the trunk seemed most ironic, if not totally appropriate: The Grateful Dead.

CHAPTER 6
THE SURGERY

In the early days of transplanting, organs were run straight into the operating room where the patient was already prepped, opened, and almost completely dissected. Sometimes guards were posted at doors to swing them open at the appointed moment. Such drama proved to be wearing on the hospital staff and disruptive to all the other surgeons counting on fresh nurses, alert anesthesiologists, and other undistracted support staff. And it soon proved unnecessary. Bo Husberg remembers a donor run in his fellowship days in Denver with Tom Starzl when the team arrived back in Denver after dawn, hopped into an ambulance and took off screaming for the hospital. Someone suggested donuts and coffee were just the elixir they all needed, and Starzl agreed. "Yes, we'll stop at the donut shop on the way in." So one block away from the donut shop, the sirens and red lights were casually turned off. The ambulance pulled in, the team got out, bought breakfast, climbed back in, and a block later, "Urrrrrrrrannnnnnnnnn" blared the ambulance, slamming on the brakes for the dramatic arrival as the liver team ran in, trying not to spill their coffee. Starzl did the same thing in Dallas with the liver for Amie Garrison that launched Baylor's program. That time, he even had a police escort.

Now, better preservation solution and quicker surgery have given transplant surgeons—and the operating room nurses and support people they rely on—the luxury of sleeping in. So even though Don Bryan's new liver was back in Dallas before dawn, the surgery wasn't started until 8:25 A.M., Sunday morning.

Pam Fertig had called Bryan the night before, 10:04 P.M., his wife, Cathy, remembered. Who could ever forget the time, the moment when the call came? Pam had not told Cathy that Don was getting the liver solely because a woman who was a closer match in size had turned it down scared or that he had lost out on another liver earlier in the day to a sixty-one-year-old alcoholic. For Cathy Bryan, who had agonized for weeks, months, over whether Don would ever get a liver in time, none of that mattered suddenly. All the pain, all the anxiety of hearing through their doctors of the transplants done each week on critical patients flown in from other hospitals and the lack of progress for Don up the waiting list, suddenly melted away. Pam's call was the call of relief, relief from changing bed pans, relief from staying up all night comforting Don, relief from dealing with a dying, confused, uncomfortable, encephalopathic grouch. With this call, Cathy had won the game of beat the clock. She had kept Don going long enough to get a liver.

The Bryans raced late that night from her sister's house in Dallas to Baylor, where they were met by Dale Distant and admitted. Don barely knew what was going on. Cathy was anxious, nervous, relieved and, now, scared. Most of the night was spent prepping Don. By six A.M., he was ready.

"We met a nice family from Midland, not far from where we live," Cathy said. "They're named Moore, and he's not doing too well the first day." It was a tough introduction to the fourteenth floor.

In O.R. 4, Tom Renard was on the lead surgeon's side; he would do the liver "skin to skin"—opening incision to closing stitches. Opposite him was Husberg, who despite the humane starting time had been at the hospital most of the previous night working on and worrying over the first transplant

■

85

of Saturday. A liver harvested from a car accident victim by Klintmalm and Caren Eisenstein on Friday had been "questionable," both from trauma damage and fat content. Quick tests were run to see if the liver was too fatty to use. The initial pathology lab findings came back borderline, but because later, permanent results always looked better than the initial quick look, Husberg decided to use the liver, transplanting it into Kelly Moore, a thirty-seven-year-old American Airlines employee. After all, Moore was in the hospital, bleeding internally, and livers were getting scarcer and scarcer. The Baylor team was consciously using livers that would have been rejected a year before, figuring that with the available drugs, the team's expertise, and the longer waiting list, they should take a shot at a marginal liver.

Husberg had done the transplant while Klintmalm was flying to El Paso Saturday morning. All had gone well, but the liver did not kick in when hooked up. It didn't start making bile, or anything else. Kelly Moore's liver-function enzyme numbers went sky high, indicating liver failure. He was dying faster than he had been dying the day before, pre-transplant. Drastic measures were under debate at his bedside.

What Husberg didn't know was that the pathology lab had changed the way it did the quick fat-content slides. A few days later, Monday afternoon, he learned that the permanent slides looked far *worse*, rather than better, under this new technique. The liver Kelly Moore got probably never should have been transplanted.

Saturday night, Husberg began debating what to do with Moore, whether to relist him on an emergency status for another liver, or perhaps whether to intercept the second liver coming back from El Paso for Moore. The liver had O-type blood, and Moore was A. Cross-matches were made in emergency cases, however. Statistically, they worked well but often resulted in more complications down the road, months out. The liver was very small, and Moore was a big guy, two hundred pounds or so. At midnight, Husberg and Klintmalm, who was finishing the second liver transplant of the day with the organ he had carried back from El Paso for the controversial alcoholic patient, began debating drastic steps as Levy was just touching down in El Paso. Maybe the thing to do was take that liver—the second one to come out of El Paso—and "piggyback" it into Moore, giving him two livers? That way, the strain would be taken off of the first transplanted liver, and it could repair itself, rid itself of all the fat and make new hepatocytes, and then the second liver could be removed.

If Moore's numbers were no better in the morning, they decided, he would get a new liver one way or another. He would probably get Don Bryan's new liver, even after Bryan had been prepped for surgery.

So instead of sleeping in, Bo Husberg was back at Baylor at 5:30 A.M., studying lab results. And the numbers were encouraging, appearing to have topped out and turned downward. Husberg decided to sit tight on Moore and give the liver to Don Bryan after all. For Don, sickly Don Bryan who everyone agreed was in dire need but had been too stubborn and proud to wait in a hospital bed, it was but another close call on the unseen liver roulette wheel.

Renard opened Bryan's skinny chest and found a liver that looked as if it had an acute case of acne, all pimply, decrepit, with brown spots and lots of white—a multicolored moonscape of craters and mountains. Renard lifted it up, and asked the "retractor-holder"—a technician who stands to the surgeon's left and keeps the metal scoop retractors that keep the chest wall pulled back and up from slipping—to grab the liver and hold it up as he worked underneath.

On a table behind the operating room, Marlon Levy was back at work, preparing the liver for the transplant. It is a separate surgical procedure—the back table work. Levy standardizes the anatomy of the new liver, correcting any defects and reworking any abnormalities in the plumbing. Ends of

■

veins are given fresh, clean edges and stretched open with tiny stitches. This brown blob of liver sits in a slush-chilled stainless steel bowl.

"Wait a minute," Renard declared, a tinge of excitement in his voice. "Can I have a pickup?"

With his loupes on, Renard delicately stretched some flesh with the pickup—a pair of tongs—and then began trimming with small scissors. Inside, he revealed a tiny vessel the width of a toothpick that had almost gone unnoticed.

"Good for you," Husberg applauded.

The mystery vessel was actually part of the arterial flow of blood to Bryan's liver. If Renard had not found it and hooked it up with the standard arteries, blood flow to the right lobe of the liver would have been cut off.

"It would have died," Renard said later. "And then we'd all go, 'What happened?'"

For Renard, this was the second liver he had done skin to skin. A Dallas native who went to Southern Methodist University in Dallas and then to the University of Texas Southwestern School of Medicine in Dallas, Renard is something of an oddity in the ranks of transplant surgeons—a born-again Christian. Cautious by nature and careful in picking his words, the sandy-haired father of two is married to a pediatrician. He had been doing a pediatric transplant fellowship at Children's Medical Center in Dallas when the head of the program suddenly walked out. Renard was left to handle the clinical care of patients while parents screamed in his face about the collapse of the program and the danger to their children. It was one of those experiences that can only be chalked up to "character building." When he was able to hold his head above water and tread for a bit, Renard called Goran Klintmalm and asked if he needed any fellows. Klintmalm was eager to rescue the young surgeon.

Casually in control now in O.R. 4, the baby-faced Renard, dubbed by some patients "Robin" to the taller Lars

Backman's "Batman," sought a change of music, as is the lead surgeon's prerogative. He asked that an Amy Grant CD be summoned from his personal music bag and cued up in the stereo.

Somehow, Christian music in this miracle factory seemed nakedly out of place. Patients talk constantly about "putting it in the hands of the Lord," or, "I turned it over to God." They place their faith, and their fate, in their religion at moments of crisis. And the hospital, a Baptist institution, lays on heavy doses of religion. The chaplain visits every patient before the transplant surgery, sometimes not knowing whether to prepare the family for life, or for death, and is a visible and integral part of the transplant team. Sometimes, though, it seems all contradictory.

To the surgeons, blind religious faith can ring hollow. They have seen too many bad things happen to too many good people, with no theological, or even medical, explanation. They create miracles on an almost daily basis, miracles that are usually the result of surgery and treatment, drugs, organ donation, and years of research and schooling. And each week they face the pressure of holding someone's fate in their hands, not God's.

It's not sacrilege, not that they don't have their own personal religious beliefs. It's just that O.R. 4 is a hard place to be a believer, an uncertain place to wear your faith on your sleeve. Songs about God often are scoffed at. But Tom Renard's Amy Grant CD, about someone going to heaven tonight, about angels and God, seemed as comfortable in the O.R. as a hen in a den of foxes.

In O.R. 4, "God" usually has a Bovie in his hand.

Don Bryan's new liver was now hooked up, filled with blood and ready to go. Husberg called for the probes to measure flow inside the hepatic artery, a clamp-like grabber placed over the artery and hooked to an electronic box that delivers a numeric readout.

101. 103. 97. 102.

■

Nothing close to the readings over 800, even 1,000, that they customarily get.

"What's wrong here?" Husberg asked innocently, as if someone other than he might have the answer. "The flow feels great in my hand."

Another probe was tried as Renard agreed that the flow looked great. Bryan's artery, tiny, curved, and stitched together like a patchwork tunnel, was pulsating with each beat of the heart, twitching back and forth like a metronome.

103. 129. 110. 150. 133. 175. 107.

"It certainly is a very small liver. But that really is a very poor rate," Husberg pondered, his bushy eyebrows furled above his demi-glasses.

"His pulse is OK," an anesthesiologist suggested.

"It certainly looks pretty," a nurse chimed in.

Husberg removed the probe, and the flow reading jumped to 450.

"Oh, wow," the anesthesiologist exclaimed, staring at the machine, not the patient. "Hold it right there."

"I took it off," Husberg said. "It reads 450 when I take it off. What is going on here?"

After a moment, Husberg pronounced Bryan fit. "The liver looks good, the artery feels good, and the machine goes to 450 when I take it off. So we're not going to worry about it, and we will measure it again at the end of the case."

Once again, it is a situation calling for Marlon Levy's favorite saying: "Better is the enemy of good." In transplant surgery, you can get into trouble trying for perfection when good will do just fine. So delicate are the moves that getting too cute can get you into big trouble.

With a needle, the portal vein was punctured and pressure was measured. (The artery, holding far more pressure, can't be punctured the way a vein can.) It checked out. Time to stitch up the bile duct, but the chatter still centered on the hepatic artery mystery.

■

"One-seventy-five is probably OK for a liver this size," Husberg said, ready to compromise and rationalize.

"It got there once, but it didn't stay long, Dr. Husberg," an anesthesiologist reminded Bo, then returned to the Sunday newspaper magazine he was reading.

Renard inserted a tiny rubber T-tube into Bryan's bile duct at the anastomosis. The tube, with one branch of the T extending into Bryan's native bile duct and the other up into the donor bile duct, helps keep the delicate biliary system open and flowing as it all heals from the surgery, and it creates a drain so that bile production, and quality, can easily be measured in the first few days after surgery. The T-tube stays in place some ten to twelve weeks, a piece of plastic hanging out of the side of the belly through a hole rather unceremoniously punched by a pair of scissors at the end of the operation. Then the rubber tube is simply pulled out. Some come out easily. Some produce leaks, resulting in incredible pain and hospitalization. One woman had a stroke shortly after Lars Backman pulled her T-tube out. Probably a coincidence, but "stroke" became one of the more talked-about complications of a T-tube pull. Among the fellows, a successful T-tube removal is something to brag about. An unsuccessful pull is a source of ridicule for weeks to come. One refrain when things are going badly: "Life sucks, and then they pull your T-tube."

With Husberg at the controls, the flow probe was placed back on Don Bryan's suspect hepatic artery.

320. "Don't touch it!" 327. 350. 337. 329. 345. 339.

"It looks better. Call it 340."

"That's OK," Husberg said. "If it had stayed very low, I would have started to talk about taking the anastomosis apart and redoing it or putting a graft in the artery—but only if it was a measurement I trusted. He has a great pulse here. It really feels alright."

Bryan's belly was X-rayed for leaks in the bile ducts, and although there was a weak-looking area on the north side of where the T-tube went in, Husberg pronounced that "I think it looks OK." After this transplant, he was scheduled to bring another patient into the OR to have a leak in his bile duct fixed. But now, it was off to give Cathy Bryan an update.

"Well, that was a nice easy case," he said at 1:30 P.M., taking off his surgical mask after a six-hour transplant.

As he has many, many times before, Bo Husberg strode swiftly to the fourteenth floor nurses' station and asked what room the Bryan family was in.

"Hello. Yes, I am Dr. Husberg. All went well, it was very good, there were no problems."

Cathy Bryan smiled with relief.

"He will be slow to wake up and will be in intensive care for a few days. He will need a lot of support from you in the coming days. But if there is one night you can take off, it is tonight. You probably should go sleep somewhere tonight. It takes a long time to wake up from surgery this long," Husberg lectured.

Cathy, intense, studious, and careful, hung on Husberg's every word. Again and again, she asked if it went well, just wanting Husberg to repeat his simple refrain: "Yes, all went well."

The family wanted more answers, but there are no others to give. It can be unsatisfying, for the reality is that the battle has just been engaged, not won. The fight is yet to come. Whether Don Bryan will survive is not clear today, only that the gods have been put off, for now.

"He said it all went well," Cathy Bryan kept repeating, no sign of worry about what may lie ahead in her voice, only the wonder of receiving good news. "I better start making phone calls . . ."

■

CHAPTER 7
THE SYSTEM

D on Bryan got a liver in time, but not everyone does at Baylor. Shortly after Bryan's transplant, Rex Voss missed his chance.

Voss was a forty-one-year-old Mississippi native who worked for Foremost Dairy Company. Divorced and remarried, he and his second wife, Kathy, had a family of four teenage boys. Bearded, good-looking, and easygoing, Voss was shown in family snapshots sitting in backyard lawn chairs, friends and a cold beer usually at hand, like some typically American fun-loving commercial scene, the ones saying, "It doesn't get any better than this."

Somewhere along the way, Voss contracted hepatitis C. No one could figure out where he got it. Many received the hepatitis C virus through blood transfusions before there was a test to detect it in the supply of donor blood. Transplant programs see patients all the time who had surgery several years previously, only to find out later they had been infected with a worse disease as a result of the earlier fix. But Rex had never had surgery and never had received blood. Regardless of the mystery, the virus, easier to transmit than the AIDS virus, had just about killed his liver. His gastroenterologist in Jackson, Mississippi, sent him to Baylor, as he had several other liver patients. Klintmalm's results couldn't be beat, he told Rex.

■

Besides, Mississippi happened to be the only state in the continental United States without a liver transplant program.

Voss arrived at Baylor in October. Rather than bemoaning his fate, he told a support group one day how lucky he felt that his employer, who had hired him just a few months before the severity of his illness was recognized, not only promised to maintain his health insurance for him but also guaranteed continued full salary. "They've been wonderful to me," he said. Not all are as lucky. The insurance horror stories often fill support group meetings.

Voss was evaluated, interviewed by Klintmalm, and accepted. After his insurance coverage was confirmed, he was placed on the waiting list and sent to his mother's home in Shreveport, Louisiana, only half as far from Dallas as Jackson. Klintmalm suggested that waiting closer would ensure Voss wouldn't miss out on a liver by being too far away.

When it comes to selecting a transplant program, patients now often have a choice: Go to a local program with less experience but more convenience or set off for a program with a national reputation and higher success statistics. Most patients assume, incorrectly, that there is one "waiting list" and that the wait for a liver does not depend on what hospital you select. For most, it is a question of excellence over convenience—some people always chase "the best" for extensive medical treatment such as a transplant, others seek the "convenience" of being close to home, others simply stay where they are, unable to even ponder negotiating the medical maze in search of other choices.

Rex Voss, more than most, was an educated medical consumer. He had studied the success statistics and heard about differences in waiting time. He had considered a program in Shreveport run by a Klintmalm trainee. Some patients in Shreveport had gotten livers after only a week or two, but Voss, still able to get around on his own and live at home, decided to go for the expertise of the Baylor program. "You don't know what to do," said his mother, Mary Jo Voss. "All the doctors we talked to said to go with the numbers."

But as his wait dragged on, his condition deteriorated. His liver wasn't producing coagulants, so he had to be hospitalized in Shreveport, then Dallas, for uncontrollable nosebleeds. Like Don Bryan, being in the hospital raised his priority—to no avail. For a time, he and his mother lived in a mobile home in the Baylor parking lot, hoping for a liver before it was too late. They didn't know the Bryans, but both families had the same wait, the same agony, at virtually the same time.

During Thanksgiving week, Voss was wheeled to the intensive care unit and placed on emergency status. His arms and legs were so weak they turned mushy. His kidneys began to fail. "What can you do?" his mother wondered later. "Maybe we should have stayed in Shreveport."

Bob Goldstein told Mary Jo that Rex would be listed for nationwide priority, "status four," likely to die soon, the highest status. Patients believe that makes them first in the nation for the next liver. Hardly. It makes them first in the nation for the next liver turned down by somebody else. Few are turned down. They may be first in priority within their local organ bank, but national sharing is an increasing rarity.

The Baylor team already had a patient in intensive care who was the same blood type, the same "status four," who would get the first available liver, Goldstein told Rex's family. Another patient came into the ICU soon after Rex—third in the emergency priority line.

At one time, a liver would probably have been available within a day for Rex. But now several factors were working against him. The nation's organ shortage is getting worse and worse. More patients with more diseases are candidates for transplants, and the number of donors is flat, at best. Seatbelt and helmet laws play a role, but families in America—for whatever reason—just don't seem to donate organs at the pace needed. Public opinion polls indicate overwhelming support for organ donation, but when families actually have to make the decision for real, they don't agree to donate organs at nearly the rates Gallup predicts. Thus the supply comes nowhere near to meeting the demand in this country. Statistics show that thousands die each year waiting.

But there's another reason why critically ill patients die waiting for organs these days, a reason even more seemingly simple to correct, yet a reason rooted in ambition and money and politics. Even though Congress mandated national sharing of organs, it doesn't happen. Organs get used, or at least offered for use, first locally. The system was set up that way for two reasons, at least on the surface: First, donation would be encouraged if people saw organs go to neighbors and if doctors and nurses could see the fruits of their procurement efforts. The public might resist donating if the organs were just flown off somewhere else, the theory went. Second, by using organs locally, the time out of a body—the time an organ sits in fluid without a blood supply—would be reduced.

The system was established at a time when kidneys were the only organ routinely transplanted by numerous programs. For livers, and to a lesser degree hearts, a handful of regional programs dominated. For them, "local" really meant regional, and the system made sense. Waits were measured in weeks, and for the most part, there were more than enough donors for the waiting transplant patients.

Now, two things have happened: Transplant programs have popped up all over, and improved preservation solutions have dramatically lengthened "ischemia time"—the time an organ will survive without blood outside the body. Livers can last up to twenty-four hours, kidneys thirty-six. (Hearts still have only a four- or five-hour window.) Yet the local-first rule has not shifted; in fact, it is more weighted locally than ever, producing a wide disparity in waiting lists. Patients at Baylor routinely wait five or six months now. Patients at smaller, less experienced programs sometimes wait just two weeks. A liver perfect for a critically ill patient in one part of a state, or even on one side of the city, might go to someone far healthier who happened to be at a hospital served by a different organ bank. It's a question of geography: Patients don't realize it, but where they are may have more to do with determining when they get an organ than how sick they are. The nation has sixty-nine different organ banks, each with its own waiting list or lists and its own set of rules. When an organ bank gets a liver, it offers it first to programs in its local service area. If no surgeon wants it there, it is then usually offered to the regional and national waiting lists.

At the time Rex Voss needed a liver, one his size and blood type might have been available—and in fact was available—but at another organ bank.

The policy has been a boon for the local programs, which now can use the supply of local livers as bait to bring in patients. Stay in Oklahoma City, you can get a liver in a couple of weeks. Go to Dallas, you may wait months.

It may not be fair and it may not even be legal. But it is a tremendous financial boon to the dozens of small transplant programs that have been started to seek a piece of what can be an incredibly lucrative and rewarding business. In the small world of transplant surgeons, pioneers and pupils all competing against each other now, the battles can be fierce, personal, and petty. The consequences can be tragic.

That was not what Congress had in mind when it created the nation's organ allocation system. The idea was to promote national sharing and to match organs equitably to those most seriously in need and who have waited the longest. But now, among those sixty-nine organ banks, competition can be intense and the goal of national sharing seems to have fallen victim to cutthroat territorialism. Since 1986, the Dallas organ bank, called the Southwest Organ Bank, has seen half its service area recruited away by LifeGift, Houston's organ bank. For hospitals, the financial incentives are enormous, not to men-

■

tion local chauvinism. Hospitals in Fort Worth, Texas, forty miles from Dallas, for example, decided to be served by Houston's organ bank. Better service, such as an organ bank coordinator on site, was one reason, they said. Another? The Houston organ bank would let Fort Worth kidney surgeons keep more kidneys for transplanting than the Dallas organ bank would. Naturally, the Fort Worth surgeons wanted more kidneys. "Despite repeated efforts to reach an accommodation with the Southwest Organ Bank, they were unwilling to allow enough kidneys to remain in Fort Worth to meet our expected transplant needs," according to Dr. Charles E. Andrews, Jr., medical director of the Houston organ bank's branch in Fort Worth and medical director of the kidney transplant program at Fort Worth's largest hospital. By having a kidney transplant program in Fort Worth, he says, the number of donors there increased from seven in the year before the program started to forty-two in 1992.

Yet the further result is that organs just next door to Dallas that might save patients such as Rex Voss are shipped to Houston, 250 miles away, regardless of the status of patients. Fort Worth patients still go to Baylor's program, but livers now go to Houston. "We see livers and kidneys and hearts go over our heads on a daily basis," Klintmalm said.

The reverse is true, too. A dying patient in Houston might miss out on a liver in Dallas, or in Galveston, a Houston-area island served by the Dallas organ bank, while the organ went to a less critically ill patient in Klintmalm's care. In fact, under the current system, "status one" patients, for whom a transplant is so early it is considered "elective," can take priority over someone in intensive care clinging to life on a respirator, simply because the two patients are in different hospitals served by different organ banks. Tom Starzl calls it "beeping patients off the golf course."

"It has come to be that the indication for liver transplantation is possession of a liver, not the need for one," fumes

■

Starzl, who says seventy percent of the patients transplanted at Pittsburgh now wait so long that they, like Rex Voss, are on life-support machines before they ever get near the operating room.

So instead of one national waiting list, there are actually sixty-nine, and really even more than that, because for some organs, hospitals within a single organ bank jury-rig their own sharing systems—rotating organs among hospitals, for example, thus bypassing the waiting list. Across the country, the rules for organ allocation vary widely and often seem screwy, founded more on what's good for hospitals than what's good for patients. Florida organ banks decided that if an organ is not used locally, it should be offered first to other *Florida* transplant programs, rather than to the national waiting list. The Dallas organ bank for years "shared" kidneys among three hospitals on a rotating basis—keep one that you procure, share the other with whichever hospital is next in line. Two organ banks serve Los Angeles: A patient at one hospital could die waiting even though a liver might be available at a hospital across town.

"The problem is there are lots of boundary lines in organ allocation. Sometimes it comes down to a street here or a street there," said Dr. Charles Miller of Mt. Sinai Medical Center in New York. "It should come down to patient status, not where it is, or who it is, which is the basis of the current system. Arbitrary geographical boundary lines force inequities."

In Rex Voss's case, a liver of the same blood type that might have saved him when he was "status four" was used in Oklahoma City, just forty minutes away by Lear jet, at a brand new program for a patient not in dire need.

"The system as it is now kills people and costs considerably more money," contends Jeffrey Romoff, president of the University of Pittsburgh Medical Center, which Starzl has built into the nation's biggest transplant center. "The patient gets the worst end of the deal."

Romoff contends the system kills people by giving some

a transplant *before* they really need it and others by denying a transplant *when* they really need it. A liver patient in relatively good shape, who could wait another year with perhaps a ninety-percent chance at survival, actually is worse off, statistically, with a transplant and now has only an eighty-percent chance of surviving the coming year. And if another patient in worse shape has to wait until consigned to the ICU, that patient's survival chances have fallen to maybe fifty percent instead of seventy percent or so. What's more, the policy leads to higher costs: The longer patients wait, the bigger the bills from the ICU before the transplant, and, if they survive, the bigger the bills after the transplant as a result of longer recovery times.

Today's system for organ distribution evolved from 1984 legislation pushed through by then-Senator Al Gore, Jr., to deal with a shortage of organs available for the rapidly emerging field of transplantation. The "Gore bill," as it became known, was meant to ensure that the sickest patients were treated first and that organs weren't allocated on the basis of financial gain. The United Network for Organ Sharing (UNOS), a nonprofit group in Richmond, Virginia, won a Department of Health and Human Services contract to run the national program. Its charge: distribute organs "equitably among transplant recipients according to established medical criteria."

By 1990, Starzl's world-famous Pittsburgh program was capturing most of the headlines for its daring breakthroughs, and capturing a huge share of the livers. The program, of course, had the lion's share of the nation's liver patients as well. The Pittsburgh machine was doing more than 600 transplants a year. It had its own fleet of aircraft to transport harvest teams. Patients were spread over four floors of intensive care beds and numerous wards. More than 100 fellows kept the seemingly chaotic program churning. Research bubbled out, paper after paper. And patient success was astounding. Despite handling some of the most difficult and challenging cases in the world, despite the risks involved in advancing the boundaries of medical technique and understanding and sometimes failing, Pittsburgh had higher one-year survival rates—seventy percent and up—than the national average.

Many of the organs were finding their way to Pittsburgh through UNOS/STAT, an emergency classification that funneled organs to dying patients such as Rex Voss, named for the hospital term for "as soon as possible." If there was a UNOS/STAT patient, a liver could be shipped off to the dying patient before it was offered to the local hospital, as long as the local patients were not in critical condition and could wait a bit longer.

But organ banks began noticing that the livers they shipped off for UNOS/STAT patients sometimes ended up in other patients. Suspicions grew that Pittsburgh was playing games with patient classification, putting some on UNOS/STAT status simply to channel livers in, then using the organs as Pittsburgh doctors wanted. If it happened, Pittsburgh people say, it was only for the good of their patients.

At the same time, regional centers were becoming more active and were finding it harder to get livers for their patients. Waiting lists were getting longer because more diseases could be treated with transplantation and more insurers were willing to pay for it. The animosity toward perceived "cheating" by Pittsburgh was growing, too, along with a tinge of professional jealousy. In time, the regional centers began feeling competition from smaller hospitals quick to get in on a good thing. All in all, it was getting harder to get livers.

In 1991, a UNOS committee of twelve transplant surgeons set in motion a subtle change in the way the nation distributes livers. The committee, which passes on recommendations to a full UNOS committee and then in turn to the full thirty-two-member UNOS board, eliminated UNOS/STAT—in effect giving even more weight to local waiting lists and further stacking the deck against patients such as Rex Voss.

The committee also voted to put in place strict qualifications for "status four" patients, allowing UNOS to make spot checks and requiring certain levels of lab results to prevent cheating. There was also a time limit on how long someone could be listed as "status four." All but one on the liver subcommittee were disciples of Starzl, including Klintmalm and Miller. Mindful of the personalities involved, a delegation was dispatched to Pittsburgh to talk with Starzl, who was recovering from his own open-heart surgery. Whether he protested then or not is a matter of debate: He says he did, others say he did not. Since UNOS was created, however, Starzl has always been a vocal advocate for a national system of sharing—one waiting list, no games or gimmicks. Just give the organs to the sickest and to those who have waited the longest. Don't punish people for their choice of surgeon, he says. Regardless of whether Starzl protested to his friends, the change was approved by the liver subcommittee, other UNOS committees, and the organization's board of directors. It never received federal approval, never received much notice at all. The public policy was made by people who ultimately may have the best of intentions and may be representing the best interest of patients, but who on the face of it, critics say, had a tremendous conflict of interest. They make policy that affects their livelihood, their practice, their hospitals. "You can't find substantive input in UNOS from the people to whom the organs are directed," says Starzl.

Charles Fiske, who served on the UNOS board after stepping into the national spotlight with a public plea for a liver to save his daughter Jamie ten years ago, came away from UNOS jaded. "The people who control the system are not the ones that depend on it for survival," he said. "They depend on it financially. . . . The fox-in-the-chicken-coop analogy does have some merit."

The 1991 change may have been subtle, but its impact has been sweeping. The result has been to benefit the fledgling local programs at the expense of the established centers. Liver transplants have exploded in the past handful of years, increasing tenfold from 308 in 1984 to more than 3,000 in 1992. The number of centers has also skyrocketed, tripling between 1988 and 1992 to 158. Yet patients have not been spread out proportionately—they chase the best care, naturally. Since patients still flock to those with the best records and reputations, the waiting lists grow and grow because the organs don't follow the patients. In livers, according to UNOS statistics, seventeen percent of the programs do sixty-four percent of the transplants. Five programs did nearly forty percent of the transplants in 1992. And thirty-two centers did fewer than ten transplants each that year. Yet those small, local programs get priority in allocations.

The pain in Pittsburgh from the allocation change was immediate and profound. Almost overnight, the number of transplants fell from 650 per year to 359. And more people are dying at Pittsburgh while waiting. Forty-six people died waiting for a liver the year before the policy change. The year after, the number had almost doubled to ninety-one. "In my mind, it can only be explained by the allocation system," says Romoff.

Frighteningly, the same thing appears to be happening nationally. In 1992, after the policy change, 492 people died while on a liver waiting list, forty-nine percent more than the 330 deaths in 1989, according to UNOS statistics. UNOS points out that the whole liver waiting list grew at an even faster pace, much faster, too, than the growth of donors, which is even falling in some areas. But critics of UNOS say the number of deaths doesn't have to skyrocket if the livers are going to the sickest patients. If the relatively healthy patients at the small centers waited a bit longer, they say, fewer people would die at the large centers like Pittsburgh and Dallas.

Starzl takes it all very personally. "It bugs the hell out of me to see something I spent my life creating turned into a piece of merchandise," he snapped. And he has considerable support from those outside the transplant programs who have benefited by the change.

"The intent of the whole effort was that organs don't belong to surgeons, they belong to the public," said Dr. Olga Jonasson of the American College of Surgeons, who led a national transplant-policy task force in 1986. "Do equally sick patients have equal chance of getting an organ?" she asked. No. The task force's answer, she said, was a national program of sharing. "It's regrettable that a national system is being bypassed without sanction by UNOS," Jonasson said.

Fiske, who now runs a Ronald McDonald–type home for transplant patients near Boston, has remained a patient-advocate as he has cherished watching his daughter, soon to be a teenager, grow with her transplanted liver. In 1993, he testified before a congressional committee examining organ allocation and distribution:

"A majority of the members of the board [of UNOS] have a direct financial interest in the future of organ transplantation and, in fact, are setting policies that control and govern their own specific institution," he said. "UNOS must be required to include a sizable number of patient/family members—consumers on its board of directors."

At the same hearing, the General Accounting Office, Congress's investigative arm, released a study of organ transplantation that put even more pressure on UNOS. The study concluded that inequities in the nation's organ allocation system deny organs to sicker patients and may violate federal law.

"Patients cannot be assured that organ procurement organizations are making equitable allocation decisions based on medical criteria," the study said.

■

The GAO focused its probe on a narrow piece of the allocation puzzle: the banks that rotate organs among several waiting lists within a single organ bank. In some cities, kidneys, for example, are shared on a rotating basis. Others have arrangements where hospitals can "keep" organs they procure in their own emergency rooms. The GAO said those types of arrangements serve specific hospitals, rather than specific patients. And that, the agency suggested, could mean a relatively healthier patient on a transplant waiting list at one hospital would receive an organ while a sicker patient nearby, but at a different hospital, would be passed by. As a result, some patients may "miss their chance," the GAO said.

The GAO said it found such arrangements at twenty out of fifty-three organ banks that serve more than one transplant center and said unless the deals were made on medical criteria, they would violate the "Gore bill"—the 1984 National Organ Transplant Act, which mandated equitable national sharing of organs. "Favoring transplant centers over the needs of patients is contrary to federal law," the GAO said.

UNOS responded by saying it was establishing a new policy requesting that organs be allocated within each organ bank on a single waiting list based on medical criteria. The new policy would eliminate special relationships with individual hospitals within each organ bank's service area. The issue of national sharing of organs was left unaddressed. What's more, UNOS also noted that its policies are voluntary, and organ banks can request waivers to the policy. If an organ bank decided to adopt a variance in defiance of the organization, "UNOS would be powerless to stop it," a UNOS statement said.

All it takes to avoid following UNOS rules is writing a nasty letter. The group admits it is bullied all the time.

"Because UNOS presently cannot enforce [organ bank] network policies, its influence has been diminished," the GAO also noted.

The GAO report also faulted the Department of Health

■

and Human Services for not monitoring and assessing organ bank practices. And the report said UNOS and HHS were not doing enough to increase organ donation.

In addition, the GAO criticized organ banks for not documenting why some patients were "skipped over" for organs and for altering UNOS criteria. Eleven organ banks adopted variances without UNOS's approval or knowledge, the GAO said, and little evaluation of the impact of the changes was undertaken. The nation's sixty-nine organ banks also have broad discretion on the condition of donors they will accept. Maximum age, for example, ranges from sixty years to ninety, the GAO said.

The GAO recommended that the government increase oversight of organ allocation, improve effectiveness of procuring organs, require organ banks to use standard criteria for ranking patients, use a single list for allocating organs within each organ bank, and document reasons for passing over higher-ranked potential recipients.

"This law has been floundering," said Representative Henry Waxman, a California Democrat, in a telephone interview the day the report was released. Waxman chairs the House Subcommittee on Health and the Environment, which held hearings on reauthorization of the National Organ Transplant Act. "I think there has been a failure to establish clear-enough standards that everyone will agree are as reasonable and fair as possible," he said.

Waxman's top aide, Michael Hash, who is something of an expert on organ donation himself, said the GAO report was one of the strongest he had ever seen. "This is an activity not being managed very well, and the oversight that is supposed to be going on is in limbo," said the aide, a senior staff associate to the House Subcommittee on Health and the Environment. "Unfortunately, this erodes public confidence. The one factor you don't want to squander is public confidence and adversely affect people's interest in being organ donors. It's terribly

■

important to reestablish a sense of direction and a sense of leadership."

Organ banks argue that local arrangements promote cooperation among competing hospitals and surgeons. The system, Stephen Haid, president of the Association of Organ Procurement Organizations, said in testimony before Waxman's committee, must be flexible enough to accommodate size and geographic variation "to promote equity among transplant patients while also balancing utility with cost and outcome."

The GAO report came three weeks after a front-page *Wall Street Journal* story detailing some of the organ allocation issues, policies, and pitfalls. The reaction was quick and sharp, pushing what had been almost "private" issues in the rather insular world of transplantation into the national spotlight. Between the story and the hearing, pressure intensified in Washington for action on the organ allocation issues.

Then along came the governor of Pennsylvania, Robert P. Casey, who checked into Starzl's Pittsburgh program for evaluation for a liver transplant. The sixty-one-year-old governor suffered from amyloidosis, a genetic liver disorder that makes the heart weak and stiff through a buildup of protein in blood. He had suffered a heart attack in 1987 and underwent quadruple bypass surgery. Six feet two, his weight had fallen to 155 pounds from 230. Starzl's team concluded that Governor Casey's heart was too weak to withstand a liver transplant, a not-all-that-uncommon fate for patients trying to get through evaluation. But the team decided to try giving the governor a heart and a liver—something Pittsburgh had attempted on only four other patients. The only one to survive more than a couple of months was Stormie Jones, a young Texas girl, who was the first person to ever receive a combined heart-liver transplant. She died five years after her Valentine's Day, 1984, operation.

Casey was put on the waiting list Sunday, and a donor

was found within twenty-four hours. On Monday, he had his double transplant, prompting an outpouring of public anger that the governor got preferential treatment. It was an ironic twist considering Pittsburgh has been most vocal in its waiting list complaints and has perhaps the longest wait of any center in the country. People in Pittsburgh ripped up donor cards. Waiting-list patients cried at support group meetings. Reporters profiled patients still waiting for organs, who might have been saved by the organs that went to the governor. UNOS tried pointing fingers at Pittsburgh, saying the actions of Starzl's team violated "national policy." Good grief. What national policy? Pittsburgh fought back, pointing out that UNOS had no policies that applied to the situation. Eventually, some new policies were proposed that would require multiple-organ transplant patients to wait on lists for each of the organs they needed.

But the public and the press—consumed with the controversy for a week or so—all missed the point. Casey jumped ahead of everyone else because he needed two organs—a standard practice at transplant centers. The organs have to come from the same donor, and finding the right donor can be difficult. The more important question that was not being asked is why the governor was up for a double transplant anyway? Would all those who were turned down because they couldn't get cardiac clearance—because, like the governor, their hearts were too diseased to survive a liver transplant—have been offered a new heart and a liver if they had been governor? Where is the wisdom of taking a dying sixty-one-year-old and, amid the crisis of the organ shortage, running the risk of wasting organs that might save two other patients, both with better chances at survival? Was this one more example of Starzl playing God, stretching the limits and stepping into yet another public firestorm? Or was this a humanitarian attempt to save a life and an important medical experiment that might save others?

■

Starzl says the governor's situation was different from all those others turned away by poor cardiac function because the heart trouble was caused by his liver disease. Cure the liver disease and the governor would not have cardiac disease—if he got a healthy heart as well. "The only difference is that if the governor had been Joe Jones, he might not have been acceptable because he couldn't pass the wallet biopsy," Starzl said on the telephone. (Casey was covered by a state insurance plan that did not balk at the experimental procedure, costing half a million dollars or so.) "You have to take my word for this, but I am certain that Governor Casey was at far greater risk of dying than any other patient on our list at that time."

Whether Casey lives to be eighty years old or not, he still won't provide an answer to the question of whether it was the right thing to do. How can the medical profession, and society, decide if one life is more important than two, or if, amid such scarcity, risks should be taken that might further science and provide greater life-saving answers down the road at the expense of a few lives along the way? Not even time can solve that dilemma.

By summer, Congress, reading the headlines and sensing public concern, was in the mood to crack down on the organ business. Waxman introduced legislation to force organ banks to operate under a single waiting list, to curb giving foreigners organs ahead of Americans (previous law limited to ten percent the number of organs a program could transplant into non–United States residents), and to force UNOS to beef up representation of transplant recipients and even donor-family members on its boards.

Before that, however, many surgeons, most notably many of the Starzl disciples who were part of the 1991 change, began voicing second thoughts and took to advocating a broader waiting list, like a "super-regional" system, where the nation would have only two or three waiting lists, and livers would be allocated solely by waiting time and how sick the patient is.

■

Canada, for instance, has a single waiting list, prioritized by urgency. European centers have gone to a more elaborate system of sharing, in some cases allocating organs to centers based on the number of patients they treat, so the bigger centers get a bigger share of the donor pool. "The issue is, frankly, patient fairness. That's what I have come to realize," said Klintmalm, who was pushing for change. "There is no reason why there is such disparity in waiting time. Oklahoma has a few days' wait. Why should new centers have priority for organs? Patients there should have to wait as long as here."

Another idea being touted is to set a bottom-line minimum survival rate—seventy percent, perhaps. Any center could stay in business and transplant anyone it wanted as long as it achieves seventy percent survival. The result would be to force surgeons to weed out some of the high-risk cases many find objectionable and to ensure that organs were used with utility and efficiency. At the same time, hospitals that do very few transplants, and have very poor success, also would be eliminated from the transplant business under such a system. "Someone should have the power to say that no center should be doing six transplants a year," Dr. Arthur Caplan, director of the Center for Biomedical Ethics at the University of Minnesota, said in a medical journal article. "Unless a hospital can come up with a very good reason to start a program, it should be told to do something else."

Rick Hurwitz, who ran an organ bank in Virginia that got caught in the middle of a nasty legal fight between competing hospitals, is convinced the system needs to be geared toward patients, not hospitals. "The bigger area of sharing is the more ethical way of doing it," Hurwitz said. "But if you talk to any individual transplant surgeon, he's interested in helping his patient at whose bedside he is standing. He views this in a very narrow way."

Charlie Miller, the New York transplant surgeon, agrees. "It's time to stop blaming," he says. "There is growing pressure that says this is unfair. . . . I think we're at that stage where people are fed up."

Do patients in fact get beeped while they're on the golf course?

"That's true," he said.

And that's not the best thing for the patient, in terms of odds of surviving the next year?

"That's true," he said.

Yet surgeons themselves have not been able to settle a nagging question as old as wartime battlefield triage. Should the sickest patients take precedence, anyway? In an emergency, should a liver be used for a sixty-five-year-old, or even seventy-five-year-old, who has been bedridden for two years and whose chances for long-term survival wouldn't be as good as those of a forty-one-year-old like Rex Voss, or even Governor Casey? Should Voss have been moved to a higher or lower priority after falling into a coma? Should a liver go to a cancer patient who has a high probability for recurrence? Or should the limited supply of organs in fact be reserved for the "healthiest"—those with the best chance for survival?

"Transplanting the sickest first, above all else, sounds honorable, but is basically dishonorable," says Ruud Krom of the Mayo Clinic, chairman of the liver committee that initiated the allocation change in 1991. "What we did with the change was give somewhat less weight to the sickest patients so other patients could be transplanted as well. The current system accepts a certain death rate."

Byers "Bud" Shaw, a Starzl disciple who runs an acclaimed liver program in Omaha, Nebraska, says the two issues must be split. The current allocation system, he says, "sucks. It's upside down." He argues too much priority is now put on saving the critically ill, comatose patient.

"Liver transplanting used to be a heroic thing in the middle of the night. A grand experiment. Then it became a therapeutic option. Now it ought to be seen as a routine treat-

■

111

ment for liver disease, with a ninety-plus percent survival rate for one year that can cost substantially less, $125,000 down to $70,000 or $80,000.

"It's a matter of triage," Shaw said. "We have to make tough decisions. We've got to understand that not everyone can be saved. . . . It shouldn't be the goal to save someone right before they die with a heroic act. . . . What I fear more than taking the executive off the golf course for his liver transplant is the sixty-five-year-old woman in ICU who hasn't been able to get out of bed in two years and is now on a ventilator. That's a bigger waste."

Patients at Shaw's center are waiting longer and longer as well. "The only patients I get livers for now are half dead and dug up," he quips.

Many suggest that transplant surgeons at the new, small centers have too much incentive to transplant easy cases first. By maintaining a high one-year survival rate, they stand to gain more business, especially through contracts with major insurers. That sounds like fingernails scratching across a blackboard to some of the founding fathers of the profession. "As doctors, our job is not to try to achieve the best results; our job is to help the sickest patients," says John Najarian, a transplant pioneer at the University of Minnesota and editor of the journal *Clinical Transplantation.*

Small programs argue in their defense that it is better for patients and their families if they can seek treatment close to home, without having to uproot the family. Relocating costs money, means more time missed at work for relatives, and can be unsettling. And some small programs have just as good one-year survival rates as the big boys. "My personal belief is the citizens of this country have the right to competent medical care locally," says Dr. Joseph Cofer, a Klintmalm trainee who did twenty-six liver transplants in 1992 at the Medical University of South Carolina. "Send my South Carolinians back to me and I'll transplant them and take the pressure off Pittsburgh and

■

Dallas," he says, echoing the sentiments of many small-pro-
gram liver transplant surgeons. "I don't see any reason to
change the system so all the livers can go to Pittsburgh."

Adds Robert Turner, a former UNOS official who is
executive director of the Oklahoma organ bank, "Pittsburgh is
squealing very loudly ever since they realized they are not going
to remain the mecca of transplantation."

Faced with the current crisis, Klintmalm, like others,
has decided to accept livers of marginal quality. For Rex Voss,
he would even have crossed blood-group lines and size criteria
once he lapsed into coma. While such stretches place patients
at greater risk, Klintmalm has been forced to do it before and
says the results to date have been adequate. With experience,
comes knowledge of how to stretch and make it work. "We'll
take anything now," he sighs.

Some surgeons have even begun trying to use livers
from non-brain-dead casualties—people injured in car accidents, for example, with no hope of recovery. When the family
decides to "pull the plug," the victim is slowly weaned from the
respirator and allowed to die in an operating room. Within two
minutes of the pronouncement of death, organs are removed.

Meanwhile, Houston's two-year-old liver program, fed
by a more plentiful supply for the relatively small program, can
be choosier. In 1992, the organ bank discarded twelve percent
of the livers donated because they didn't meet surgeons' standards, according to Rebecca Davis, director of LifeGift,
Houston's organ bank. The donor livers rejected by Houston
were offered elsewhere, but none were accepted. Once rejected
by one set of transplant surgeons, it's hard to take a gamble and
risk the liability. Different surgeons faced with different pressures act differently for the good of their patients. And using
marginal livers can carry a risk. "We must often temper our
enthusiasm to help our critically ill patients with the realization that each transplant carries the potential for two people to
die," Dr. Patrick Wood, chief of the Houston liver transplant

program, said in response to the *Wall Street Journal* story. "Not only might the recipient of the liver die, but one of the other, less critically ill patients on the transplant waiting list who could have received the same liver may die before another liver can be located. The use of marginal livers may result in poor initial liver function and if a substantial number of patients require retransplantation, this further depletes the already limited donor pool."

UNOS officials vigorously defend the current allocation system as fair to all patients because livers must be rationed in time of shortage and because promoting local health care—small-hospital transplant programs—is the choice of the UNOS board. Dr. Randal Bollinger, UNOS chairman in 1993, argues a national waiting list would be impossible since organs have a finite life in preservation solution, although opponents of the policy argue the time has stretched to eighteen to twenty-four hours, more than enough to offer wider sharing and distribution.

"If you give livers just to all sick people, then you'd have to get sick just to get a liver," said Dr. Jeremiah Turcotte of the University of Michigan Medical Center, a member of the UNOS liver subcommittee. "You've got to have reasonable access for people. I think what you'd find if you had only ten big centers is only the upper class would get livers. We've got to reach some sort of compromise."

Compromise, though, favors those with a voting majority. And by the nature of UNOS, the small centers can outvote the major programs. "The fundamental problem with UNOS is that UNOS is a center democracy. One center, one vote," Klintmalm said. "When I left Pittsburgh I had as many votes as Tom Starzl did after twenty years in the field. We have the Senate. We lack the House. It takes only two centers doing five transplants per year to outvote Tom Starzl or Bud Shaw."

Bud Shaw agrees. "Right now, UNOS has been unable

to deal with this because it is a politically charged issue," he said.

"The real objective is maximum efficiency to patients and programs be damned," adds transplant surgeon Todd Howard of Washington University in St. Louis. "The problem is decisions are made by people running the programs, not people getting the organs, and there can't help but be some self-interest."

In addition to the questions over how to decide which patient gets an organ, there is yet another wrapped up in the debate: Which surgeons are good enough to use the limited supply of organs available? Given the shortage, why risk in the hands of the inexperienced or the incompetent a donated liver than can save a life? Among transplant surgeons, there is a growing concern that the unthinkable may have to be contemplated, the unspeakable may have to be spoken in the medical profession: The less-than-sterling performers in transplant surgery may have to be weeded out.

In 1992, the government began publishing center-by-center survival statistics for the nation's transplant programs. The numbers showed how many were attempted, how many lived, and how many died. They also tried to take into account the severity of patient illness at the time of the surgery, recognizing that a critically ill patient is more likely to die than someone beeped off a golf course, and thus one death may not be as indicative as another. So the study gave an expected survival rate for each transplant center and compared that to the actual results.

Those results, overall, showed many skilled programs do very, very well at transplantation. But the volumes of reports, which are supposed to be available to patients but in reality are little known and probably little used, also contained some horror stories. Heart transplants seemed to be the most alarming. The nation's hospitals have opened 158 different heart programs, perhaps more than exist in the rest of the world combined, even though there are only 2,000 or so heart transplants attempted annually in the United States. The number of hospitals doing heart transplants has doubled since 1985, and some cities have four and five programs from which to choose. Now, only three hospitals do more than fifty heart transplants a year in the United States; sixty do fewer than ten transplants a year, according to UNOS statistics.

The result is that only a few heart programs have enough business to build a full-time practice in what is a difficult and delicate art. For most centers, transplantation has become a sidelight to valve replacements, bypasses, and other cardiac surgical routines. Doctors find themselves inexperienced in dealing with the unique drugs, tests, and equipment of transplantation, not to mention novel physiological balances in remade bodies.

The bottom line is that the rush to glory and intense competition may actually result in more deaths and higher costs. At Kansas City's Menorah Medical Center, six of the first eight heart transplant patients died, giving the program one of the worst survival rates in the nation, while cross-town rival St. Luke's sported better than an eighty percent first-year survival rate for the same period.

In the same government report, the first to ever publish center-by-center results for transplant programs, the heart-transplant program at Humana Hospital in Louisville, Kentucky, posted a one-year survival rate of fifty percent, while Jewish Hospital in Louisville came in at seventy-six percent. Of the first ten patients who went to University Hospital in Cleveland for a new heart, five died. Would they have been better off at the large program at the Cleveland Clinic, with almost ninety percent one-year survival for the same period? That question is impossible to answer, and experts caution that the government statistics are a small, limited snapshot of data easily influenced by unfortunate events. Still, the report offers

■

patients a tool to access programs, and the public a method of raising questions about the efficacy of the explosion of transplant programs. In St. Louis, two patients ended up at suburban Depaul Health Center for heart transplants, and both died. The program was shut down, leaving only the question of whether it ever should have opened. Across town, Barnes Hospital at Washington University has a highly regarded program with success at better than the national average, and St. Louis University Hospital does even better at nearly ninety-four percent one-year survival.

Studies show that in many cases, those that do the most transplants have the best results. In livers, a different center-by-center study of survival statistics found that programs that fared particularly poorly did a very small number of procedures—six livers a year or so. Another recent study found that at hospitals with fewer than nine heart transplants a year, mortality rates were forty-six percent higher than at high-volume centers. And the disparity can be quite broad. Ten heart transplant centers have one-year survival rates below fifty percent, while thirty-two centers have survival rates above ninety-five percent, according to a federally funded study conducted by Roger Evans, a Mayo Clinic health services researcher.

"It can be like playing roulette," Evans said.

Indeed, to explain its dismal results, Menorah Medical Center pointed to the sidelight nature of its transplantation enterprise. "The cardiac transplant program is a relatively small part of the Menorah Medical Center cardiac surgery program," Dr. Hamner Hannah III assured readers of the government statistics, and "not an accurate reflection of the commitment to care and standards of excellence." Still, "this service is offered to our patients as part of Menorah's continued commitment to be on the contemporary edge of science in its cardiac program," he wrote.

Transplantation experts, even those running the system, say the nation lacks any performance standards at all.

■

UNOS has tried to enforce minimum criteria for the number of transplants a program has to do each year to stay in business, but it can't even do that. "If a veterinarian or a dentist wanted to open a transplant center, they could. That's kind of scary, I know," UNOS's communications director, Wanda Bond, said, exaggerating a bit. The minimums for the number of transplants a center has to do to have access to organs, and for the qualifications of surgeons, can't be enforced because UNOS membership is voluntary.

In livers, the one-year survival rates in the government report averaged seventy-four percent nationally, but ranged from zero to one hundred percent. Some large centers, such as Johns Hopkins University and Rush-Presbyterian-St. Luke's Medical Center in Chicago, stood out as faring poorly, and complained that they were, in essence, penalized for taking on high-risk cases or trying innovative therapies. "If you threaten centers with this sort of blanket, superficial scrutiny, you are telling them they can't afford to take care of patients with a fifty-fifty chance of survival," Dr. James Williams told a medical magazine in explaining his program's results. "You're inadvertently causing the rationing of care, and that's wrong."

But care must be rationed because of the shortage of organs. If a hospital is not as skilled in handling those fifty-fifty patients, maybe they should be sent to someone who has more success, or maybe they shouldn't be transplanted at all. The questions are difficult ones to resolve, and the choices strike at the core of our medical system: We, as a nation, abhor ever giving up on saving someone. We are also loathe to criticize our doctors, and they are equally uncomfortable with outside scrutiny.

An unlikely but possible solution may be that the government will ultimately step in. The federal government tests drugs for safety and effectiveness, but not doctors. With the shortage of organs for transplants, and now a unique wealth of survival data in that field, demands for action against the poor

■

performers may increase. At the least, the Department of Health and Human Services could make UNOS policies mandatory. Then again, if patients had both the data and the ability to make a choice and pick a hospital and surgeon without increasing the risk of dying on a long waiting list, then the free market would squeeze out the weak programs. For now, the weak programs have a crutch—the jury-rigged, localized allocation system.

Defenders of the current system also argue strongly that the root of the problem is the organ shortage—no matter how you divide up the supply of livers, there will not be enough, and someone will die. "Liver allocation is not the problem. Lack of donors is the problem," said Robert Turner, the Oklahoma organ bank director. "A national list doesn't provide more livers. The problem is the shortage of organ donors."

Yet even the organ shortage itself is a cause of criticism of UNOS. Everyone involved agrees that too many people are buried with organs that might save someone else. For whatever reason, American society is behind the times in organ donation. Other nations donate at far higher rates. Other legislatures, in Europe primarily, have gone to "presumed consent" systems—everyone's organs will be shared upon brain death unless the person had specifically expressed opposition. The rationale is that sharing is a fundamental tenet of society. Yet in the United States, the system presumes opposition to organ donation and makes it possible only if the family takes affirmative steps.

For some, organ donation may be antithetical to religious beliefs. For others, distrust and dislike of the medical establishment gets in the way. Research has found that racial issues play a role: African-Americans don't donate at nearly the level whites do, because they distrust the white-dominated medical establishment. That's especially tragic because African-Americans are three times as likely to suffer kidney disease, and the current kidney allocation systems matches tissue types, making it harder for African-Americans to receive a Caucasian kidney. The result: African-Americans, twelve percent of the population, make up one-third of the kidney waiting list.

Those specific reasons aren't what lead most to shun donation, however. For the vast majority, the question is simply far too difficult to deal with at the moment of grief. A 1993 Gallup Poll found that eighty-five percent of the American public supports organ donation and sixty-nine percent would be very willing to donate their own organs upon death. That landslide at the polls doesn't match what actually happens, however. Organ banks report that only one-third of families actually consent to organ donation. Even though a person may designate organ donation on a driver's license, those wishes won't be fulfilled in most states if any family member expresses a reservation to a doctor or nurse. No matter how slight the misgiving may be, everyone backs off. There is no pressure; nor should there be at that moment.

Since the driver's license laws have made little improvement in organ donation, some states are now trying to take further steps, such as making the wish expressed on a driver's license mandatory—incapable of being overridden by a balking family member. Some are even pondering presumed consent. And the federal government has asked Congress for a massive organ donation awareness campaign on the score of antismoking or AIDS-awareness efforts. The chances of that seem slim. The reality is that death is something we, as Americans, don't like to talk about, don't like to plan for, don't like to accept. We'll try any expensive and heroic measure to prolong life in the elderly. Mortality seems almost an un-American concept. And it's surely easier to ignore the problem than to deal with it.

Until you have to be on the receiving end.

Yet there may be some very simple answers to the problem. And that's where the gripes about UNOS and its organ procurement organizations come back in. Critics say organ banks and hospitals do a poor job of dealing with a very sensitive and difficult issue and may be ignoring some simple answers by stubbornly clinging to old, ineffective practices while defensively shrugging off new ideas.

Doctors and a nurse from an organ bank in Kentucky met with a management consultant from Boston to see if there was not a better way to handle the question of donation. The answer: Simple changes in the way hospitals approach families about organ donation can have significantly better results.

The researchers reviewed 32,562 deaths in 1988 and found 173 potential solid organ donors, but only thirty-eight actually became donors —a success rate of only twenty-two percent. The study blamed physicians for failing to recognize the potential for donation in twenty-nine instances, with the family refusing consent in ninety-two cases. Five potential donors had voiced an objection before death, and the remaining nine had died in the first few hours after arriving at the hospital and were listed as potential donors because of isolated extensive head injury. The study said if those patients had received an aggressive resuscitative effort, "all could have been salvaged for organ donation."

The next year, the Kentucky group analyzed 143 donor referrals, focusing this time on the timing of the request for donation. In eighty-two cases, the question of organ donation was put to the family *after* the explanation of death or the certainty of family acceptance of death. Fifty-three of those potential donors actually became donors—a sixty-four-percent success rate. On the other hand, in sixty-one instances where the discussion of death and the discussion of donation were *combined*, only eleven families consented—a success rate of a mere eighteen percent.

The study, published in 1991 in the journal *Surgery*, also noted that in Kentucky at the time, there were adequate numbers of potential donors available to meet the need for organs for transplant patients. The reason people were dying while waiting for organs came down to consent, not supply, and the consent issue really boiled down to a simple matter of the timing of the request.

Out of that experience, Michael Evanisko, the management consultant from Boston, who is also on the board of directors at the Harvard University School of Public Health, formed a nonprofit group called The Partnership for Organ Donation to spread the word. The partnership also sponsored the landmark 1993 Gallup poll asking how Americans felt about donation. Now, Evanisko preaches that the organ shortage is solvable if more thought and planning go into how families are approached about this delicate question. Don't have the doctor who explains brain death and delivers the bad news be the one to ask about organ donation, he says, that looks too much like a conflict. Give the family some time, for God's sake. Don't hit them with the horror, then the decision, all in the same breath. "The organ shortage exists despite the fact that there are more than enough potential organ donors to fill the current need," he says.

A 1992 study by Roger Evans, the highly respected health-care researcher then with the Battelle-Seattle Research Center and now with the Mayo Clinic, seemed to back Evanisko up. Evans, along with colleague Carlyn Orians and pioneering transplant surgeon Dr. Nancy Ascher, estimated the donor supply in the country and measured the efficiency of organ procurement efforts. What they found is that the number of donors had remained more or less unchanged from 1986 through 1990, and organ procurement efforts are between thirty-seven and fifty-nine percent efficient. "Efficiency greatly varies by state and organ procurement organization," the study, published in the *Journal of the American Medical Association*, noted. "Many more organ donors are available than are being accessed through existing organ procurement efforts," the study concluded. "Realistically, it may be possible to increase

■

by eighty percent the number of donors available in the United States (up to 7,300 annually). It is conceivable, although unlikely, that the supply of donor organs could achieve a level to meet demand." Of the twenty states with the highest numbers of potential donors, Florida, Missouri, Ohio, Pennsylvania, and Wisconsin were the most efficient in 1989; Louisiana, New Jersey, New York, North Carolina, and South Carolina were the worst.

Despite the data and studies, Evanisko is now incredibly frustrated. No one seems to be listening. A handful of organ banks have worked with his group, which now has an all-star transplant community board of directors. But UNOS, the national network, he contends, has been passive and ineffective. Doctors are reluctant to change. Hospitals can be slow to respond. People are set in their ways—they do things the same way, day after day. "The organ shortage is a public health crisis with a cure," he says. Yet, "UNOS has not been an effective manager of the donation system."

Florida stands out as an illustration that Evanisko may be right—both about the ability to solve the organ donation problem, and about UNOS being an ineffective manager. The Lifelink Foundation, the organ procurement agency serving most of Florida and Georgia, leads the nation in organs acquired per population served, and since 1989, donations have actually increased at twice the national rate. Lifelink says its success is the result of intensive programs of contact with hospital professionals; with a simple thing such as eliminating an hour's worth of paperwork for a nurse—lo and behold— nurses become more willing to participate in the organ donation process. "If every organ procurement program in the United States were performing at the level of Lifelink's Florida programs [thirty-three donors per million population], there would be virtually as many organs available for transplant as there are persons waiting on the national list," according to John R. Campbell, executive vice president of Lifelink. Such

■

efforts aren't cheap: Overhead at Lifelink is among the most expensive in the nation.

But like just about everything having to do with the complicated world of transplantation, there's more to the Lifelink story. A *St. Petersburg Times* investigation accused the nonprofit group of gross misspending, ghoulish aggressive procurement tactics, and even nepotism—putting relatives and friends with no medical background in charge of bone and tissue banks, for example. The newspaper found that Lifelink, which is based in Tampa, leases medical equipment and office space for more than $1 million a year from private firms made up primarily of some of its own directors and officers. Some of the rents paid were three times the going rate, the newspaper said. Salaries of the top five executives in 1991 totaled $548,000, and other employees received bonuses that the newspaper criticized as "bounties" on body parts. The *Times* said six employees were rewarded with a trip to Maui financially finagled to be reimbursed by Medicare—by taxpayers. Lifelink claimed it paid bonuses to the employees—and what they did with the cash was their business.

In its defense, Lifelink said it had never been investigated, and no one was unduly profiting from its arrangements. But the newspaper's stories, by reporter Jeff Testerman, threw the first half of the statement out the window by prompting a congressional investigation into organ procurement agencies and an audit of Lifelink's books. The audit by the Health Care Financing Administration found Lifelink had overbilled the federal government by $490,280 in fiscal year 1991 in categories such as office expenses, salaries, pension contributions, dues and subscriptions, a charter airline flight, and a lobbyist's fee. Lifelink appealed the finding.

UNOS says it is hard at work on the problem of organ donation consent and notes again that it is a voluntary organization that cannot dictate what procedures hospitals, or even organ banks, follow. The popular wisdom is that the organ shortage is a result of lack of public education, and UNOS, in front of Waxman's committee, pleaded for federal money for a massive organ donor awareness campaign. The GAO report, however, echoing Mike Evanisko, said UNOS and HHS weren't doing enough to increase organ donation with the resources they did have.

Maybe the bottom line is that the problem is more a result of ignorance and stubbornness in the medical community itself. Maybe over time, attitudes will change, both among the professionals on the front lines of the battle and the families who find themselves facing tough decisions amid the most unbelievable moments of hell. Maybe more light will be shed on the agencies set up to procure organs, and maybe they will improve beyond being defensive. Maybe some of the fears and taboos of organ donation will be stripped away, the misconceptions shed. Maybe the supply will someday meet demand, either because there are more donors or because cures for diseases are found that eliminate the need for radical treatments such as organ transplants. Maybe even one day, animals will be able to provide an unlimited supply of life-saving organs.

Maybe came too late for Rex Voss.

After several days of waiting, a debate began raging at Voss's bedside: Had he gone too far to transplant? The lack of livers had forced a choice: Who would live and who would die?

Rex Voss had missed his chance. He was moved to "status seven"—inactive—on the waiting list. "These smaller centers are scarfing up livers while this guy crashes and burns," bristled Bob Goldstein. "I had to tell Rex Voss's family: 'He won't be a candidate, and he will probably die.'" Mrs. Voss pleaded for another chance; Goldstein promised he would come by twice a day and check for improvement.

One other patient in intensive care did get a liver, flown in from Detroit. She recovered and returned home to south

Texas. For the two others, there was nothing to do but stand by and watch.

Rex Voss died December 8, 1992.

His obituary in the local newspaper asked people to sign up as organ donors.

CHAPTER 8
THE SUPREME COURT

llocating medical treatment has never been an easy task in the United States or in any other country. Some nations have decided to make less available but to make the basic services available to all. Such systems of "nationalized" health care, such as the Canadian or British health care systems, make many Americans bristle. The government running things? What could be more disastrous, they argue. For now at least, until true reform reshapes our health care system, we have chosen a good old American system: the dollar speaks. If you want the best health care, you have to pay for it. And if you can pay for it, you can get the best in the world. If you can't pay for it, you're shunted off to second-best, although still better than much of the world.

From time to time, there are exceptions. In the 1960s, the journalist Shana Alexander, well-known for her best-selling books and point-counterpoint arguments with Jack Kilpatrick on the CBS show "60 Minutes," went to Seattle to see how the this new wondrous technology, kidney dialysis, was functioning. What she found shocked the nation. Kidney dialysis treatment was expensive, and the dialysis machines were in very short supply. The result was that time on the machine was allocated by a selection committee, a group of men deciding who should live and who should die. Alexander's *Life* magazine account of the committee, and the often arbitrary and money-oriented decisions it made, touched off a firestorm of criticism and led Congress to fund a law making kidney dialysis available to all who need it, without racial, social, or financial discrimination.

Now liver transplanters are facing the same question that the kidney dialysis folks did thirty years earlier, perhaps even the same type of criticism. There are not enough livers for those who need them. So the recipients must be "selected"—chosen from a pool of potential candidates. The way they did with the kidney dialysis problem, hospitals have set up "selection committees" to make these tough choices—the supreme courts for the dying. As with the kidney dialysis problem, money plays a role in selecting who will get a liver and who won't. And while professionalism and strict guidelines are the order of the day, arbitrary and capricious reasoning can play a role, and issues become murky and contrived. "This guy deserves a liver," someone declares. "I don't like him," or "I don't trust him," says someone else.

Two primary rules are used to screen candidates at most hospitals, one medical, one not. First, patients must be surgically "doable." They must not have cancer outside the liver, with the possible exception of brain tumors. They must not be HIV-positive, although that "contraindication" has come under some question. They must not have an active, untreatable infection, and they must have adequate heart capabilities to withstand the operation.

Second, they must be able to pay—they must pass what Tom Starzl calls "the wallet biopsy." Some simply have to get their insurance companies to agree to the transplant, and today, more than eighty percent of private health insurers cover liver transplantation. Some patients are old enough, or poor enough, to get the government to pay, through the federal Medicare program for the elderly, or the state Medicaid program for the poor. Medicaid programs in forty-seven out of fifty states will pay for an organ transplant, according to a study from the Mayo Clinic. But the qualification for Medicaid is very, very low. In most states, a family with household income of about $7,000 per year would not qualify.

Add to that mix some thirty million Americans who are without health insurance, and the result is that at least twenty-five percent of the United States population is without health insurance or uninsured should they require an organ transplant (other than a kidney). Their only recourse is to write a check, or somehow raise $150,000 to $300,000, sometimes even through bake sales and raffles.

A few get around the rules, of course. Some patients who did not meet the federal or state guidelines for Medicare or Medicaid nonetheless have gotten a congressman or senator to badger some bureaucrat into saying "yes." Some, turned down by their insurance companies on technicalities or fine-print regulations that give the companies an out, end up fighting long enough, or hard enough, to bring about a change of corporate heart or a court judgment forcing the change of heart. Others intentionally bankrupt themselves, or divorce their spouses, in order to qualify under a payment program. Given that the alternative is death, society has forced some very grim choices on a few of its hard-luck members.

In most cases, in most hospitals, even after a patient has passed those two tests, the decision still boils down to the selection committee, a group set up to make the tough calls with whatever impartiality and objectivity they can muster. Inevitably, the criteria and the decisions become murky. Two nearly identical cases might get different votes when attendance varies, as it must, from week to week. One faction can outvote another sometimes. One forceful voice might carry the day for one patient, yet another one might be turned away because the chief of surgery did not come to argue on that patient's behalf.

And then there are all the troublesome questions that

must be answered. How old is too old? What was too old two years ago is no longer too old. For alcoholics, how sober is sober enough? Six weeks sobriety? Six months? Six years? What if the patient is within days of dying? Is he turned down simply because he has not been sober for six months?

How much should social morals play a role? The man was abusive to the inquiring social worker—should he be sent away to die? What about the young father who may be psychologically unstable? What if the patient doesn't have the necessary family support, will she die for lack of a loving companion? What about drug users? The guy who happened to test positive for marijuana in a routine blood test? People who wouldn't follow doctors' orders in the past? What about the woman who, with no other way to pay for the transplant, "divorced" her husband, quit her minimum-wage job, and impoverished herself to qualify for Medicaid? Does she get in? And what about the close friend of the hospital administrator? The close friend of the governor? Just because the governor called the president of the hospital on her behalf, should that influence the committee?

It can.

At Baylor, the liver selection committee convenes on Wednesdays in a long, brightly lit conference room, a couple of pizzas from Domino's on the table, along with an ice bucket and some Diet Cokes. Patients are told a committee meets to select patients, but that's about all. The meetings are confidential so that the honesty and integrity of opinions are preserved. Nobody wants a dying patient or angry family coming after him because the doctor did not speak well of them in the selection committee.

About eight to twelve people vote each week, the number varying with attendance. There are thirteen voting members of the committee—all men, all white. Five are gastroenterologists who care for the patients before the transplant.

■

Four are surgeons—Klintmalm, Goldstein, Husberg, and Levy—who care for the patients after the surgery. Two are cancer specialists, and two others are internists not directly connected to the transplant program. Another eight or so are nonvoting members: heart specialists, a psychiatrist, two social workers who evaluate each patient, a chaplain, a financial services administrator. Coordinators sit in, fellows sit in, research nurses sit in. The overriding objective is to pick the patients for whom transplants can result in an improvement in the quality of life. There's the rub: It's a judgment call almost every time. Selection committee is Judgment Day. There are no representatives of the public, no pure patient advocates. Dale Distant, the fellow from New York, believes the committee should not be operating in secrecy, that there needs to be a "societal" representative. Maybe there should be a mother or two, maybe a genius, or a laborer, or a political or business leader with decision-making prowess. Without someone from the outside, the committee's doings may come under suspicion.

As in any group, there are alliances, voting blocs, and personal relations. The nonvoting chief cardiologist happens to be married to one of the gastroenterologists. A couple of the committee members date others in the room. The psychiatrist happens to be the brother-in-law of one of the surgeons. If everyone is there, the transplant surgeons can be easily outvoted—their program is out of their control. The exchanges can become quite heated.

The committee is chaired by Dan Polter, the longtime and revered head of Baylor's gastroenterology department. He is the quiet voice that roars when he talks, always softly, always sparingly, always deliberately, always on target. Like a grandfather presiding over a rancorous Thanksgiving family reunion, Polter will let a discussion bounce back and forth with passion, then quietly inject a thought not previously raised, often cutting the argument to the quick.

The meeting begins with a review of "the service"—the status and condition of liver transplant patients in the hospital. One day Polter asked Klintmalm for "the sermon," as opposed to the service. Taking the opening, Klintmalm preached about the merits of this patient or that case, concluding with "Amen."

"Amen" seemed much more appropriate in the formal setting where the committee is playing God than the sterile operating room dominated by the hands and fingers of the surgical gods.

Each patient's case is presented by his or her gastroenterologist, or at least by that doctor's assigned fellow. Technically, this is the one person in the room who is the patient's advocate. An evaluation package is distributed containing the patient's history, important lab results, and one-sentence summaries of the various evaluations by radiology, pathology, the kidney specialists, the transplant surgeons, the psychiatrist, and the cardiologists.

Once the presentation is done, Polter goes around the room. Cardiology says he is an acceptable candidate. Ditto for the transplant surgeons. Social work says he is OK. Everyone agrees, this guy needs a liver, is a good candidate, and will be put on the list. No discussion needed.

Of the hundreds of cases presented to the Baylor committee each year, that is the routine. The situations are usually clear-cut: either the patient is "in" medically, or "out" medically.

But there are disagreements. For the tricky cases, the committee agonizes. It is forced by medical society to operate with no guidelines, and forced to be responsible custodians of a limited resource. Much of the angst stems from efforts to make decisions as objective as possible. "We struggle so very hard to make sure we give every patient a fair chance," Klintmalm said. "We try as best as we humanly can to not make arbitrary decisions. And we agonize every time, because we know we are condemning patients to death." As hard as they try, though, the bottom line to some choices is, "Does he *deserve* a liver?" How can you decide who deserves a liver? The committee has a job that sometimes seems impossible.

The day before Thanksgiving, two nearly identical patients came before a selection committee thinned out by vacation. Chuck Palmer, a twenty-three-year-old cook in the National Guard from Seattle came to Baylor with a huge tumor in his liver. He had had the tumor for more than a year and a half, and the army doctor, like many in the medical profession, had driven a wedge-like biopsy device into the tumor to remove a chunk and make sure it was cancer. The problem with "wedge biopsies" is that the tumor bleeds, and the cancer cells are then scattered throughout the belly, seeded as it were. Baylor sees cancer patients come in all the time after wedge biopsies. What did the original physician think the huge growth on the liver was? Of course it was cancer. Why bother seeding it all through the abdomen, helping it spread?

As much as they liked Chuck Palmer, the wedge biopsy to some seemed to guarantee that the tumor had spread. Once he got a transplant and his immune system was suppressed, the cancer would take off and would surely kill him. Quickly. There was no point in doing the transplant.

On Palmer's evaluation sheet, a cancer specialist noted that a computer-enhanced scan and a sonogram already suggested the cancer was visible beyond the liver—a mass was seen elsewhere. "It appears that he is not an acceptable candidate for transplant," the oncologist concluded before heading off to grandma's home for Thanksgiving. But Daniel DeMarco, Palmer's gastroenterologist who, as much as anyone, takes his role as patient advocate to heart, announced to the committee at the start of the meeting that the oncologist had changed his opinion after further tests found that the mass was actually blood, not cancer, and had been removed. "Give him the benefit of the doubt then," the oncologist was quoted by DeMarco as saying on the telephone from Waxahachie.

Sentiment began swinging in Palmer's favor. Someone noted that by the time Palmer gets a liver, there would be a reasonably good chance that the surgeons could see if there were "metastases"—areas where the cancer had taken root. Do him with a backup, and give the kid a shot. Someone else suggested sending him to chemotherapy first, zapping the tumor and its seeds, and then transplanting him. "That doesn't work," someone else said bluntly, ending that approach.

Klintmalm, who had come in during a week of vacation to the selection committee in jeans, black boots, and a silver belt, began voicing concerns along with other surgeons. Palmer's lymph nodes looked as if he already had cancer that had spread. The wedge biopsy could not be ignored, it was like a death sentence for the kid. The waiting list had grown to fifty-three, and the wait was topping five months. Shouldn't all the others—people with a better chance of survival—be factored in here, too? The committee had to realize that it had to make tough choices. And there was something else at stake— Klintmalm's cancer research. He was on the verge of publishing results of his protocol, which showed great promise in treating liver cancer. If the committee took a patient destined to die, then the results of the Klintmalm protocol would be skewed, hurt. A life-saving treatment that might be adopted around the world and prove to save thousands of people might end up in the scientific dumpster because of terminal patients such as Palmer who hurt the success numbers and discouraged others from trying the protocol. So far, he had achieved fifty percent survival for four years—multiples better than any other treatment for these tumors. There was a lot at stake, something more important than one patient, even a nice twenty-three-year-old from Seattle stricken with the worst kind of luck.

■

"I wish Marvin Stone was here," someone said, referring to the chief cancer specialist at Baylor, a voting member of the committee.

Just then Marvin Stone walked in, as if on cue. If there was seeding, he opined, then the Klintmalm chemotherapy protocol might handle it. If they couldn't find cancer outside the liver now, then the kid might be all right. Stone spoke favorably of Palmer. Give the guy a shot, he suggested.

Time to vote. All those in favor of accepting Charles Palmer? Four "yes" votes. Opposed? Five "no" votes. Palmer was rejected.

"This Wednesday afternoon massacre will continue," Polter declared. Next up was an almost identical case, Kirstan Reading, a thirty-five-year-old woman from Florida with a huge solid tumor in her liver. She had been sent to New Orleans to have the tumor surgically removed, but once doctors got to it, they found it was impossible to cut it all out. They closed her back up, but first took a wedge biopsy. Yup, cancer all right. Then, out of options, she was sent to Baylor for a transplant. There was no evidence that the cancer had spread outside the liver, but there again was the question of the wedge biopsy.

Frustration was rampant. How, someone asked, could they make life and death decisions on the limited information they had? How could they be sure, even after all the tests that had been run? How could they accept one and not the other? It was a guessing game, an exercise in agony, no other way to look at it. But lives were in the balance.

Polter took the second vote. All those in favor? Five "yes" votes. All opposed? One. Abstain? Three. She was in. Chuck Palmer was out. How could this be?

Polter quickly noted that one member had voted against Palmer, then for Reading. "Could I ask why?" he said.

"Because [the oncologist who saw Palmer] said he was

not an acceptable candidate," the voter, who had come late to the committee meeting, responded.

"REVOTE!" someone shouted. The voter was told that before he had arrived, DeMarco had explained to the committee that the oncologist had changed his opinion since the mass outside the liver had turned out to be blood, not cancer.

Polter called for a vote again on Chuck Palmer. Five "yes"es, he was in, the crucial fifth vote coming not from the late-arriving misinformed voter, but from one of the surgeons who believed that if Kirstan Reading was in, then Chuck Palmer should be in as well. There was only one vote against Palmer this time. The rest, including the late arriver, abstained.

For Palmer and Reading, it turned out to not make any difference. A later test showed that cancer had spread to Palmer's hepatic artery, making him ineligible under the program's rules. DeMarco, however, would not give up. He lobbied the surgeons in the hospital corridor: Couldn't they break the rules? This was a twenty-three-year-old kid who had no other chance, for God's sake. He was dead otherwise. What was wrong with breaking the rules?

A deal was struck. One of the surgeons would open him up and hunt for cancer. The surgeon found nothing, and Palmer got back on the list. Livers came up for Palmer and Reading within twenty-four hours of each other, the Sunday after Christmas. But both were opened and closed with no transplant. By this time, four weeks after they had been evaluated, four weeks of waiting for livers the right size and blood type, cancer had indeed spread beyond the liver. The livers went to their backups, and Palmer and Reading went home.

Few decisions were as contentious as the Thanksgiving almost-massacre, but some are. Alcoholism is a frequent cause of controversy, and age is a chronic cause of dissonance.

A sixty-nine-year-old man in terrible shape was pre-

■

sented to the committee the Wednesday before the November election, in that somber time when the transplant team struggled with several patients. The man, Roy Clover, had diseased bile ducts, which were diagnosed thirteen years earlier. He had been evaluated for a transplant a year before and was told he was not yet sick enough. Doctors kept his bile ducts open by threading metal stents—flexible strips—inside. Now, he was bedridden from his liver disease and a host of other woes, such as ulcerative colitis and heart valve problems. He was on eight different medications. One year before he had not been sick enough. Now, the question arose: Was he too sick?

Clover sailed along through the committee discussion, appearing to be on his way to routine acceptance. Then Goran Klintmalm began to speak.

"With patients over sixty-five, we have a fifty-percent one-year survival rate," he said. "That's worse than with hepatitis B."

Quickly, battle lines were drawn along the usual lines, the gastroenterology staff was eager to get its patient transplanted because they had run out of treatment options. The surgical staff was hesitant. The man was old and very sick. Recently Marlon Levy had completed a study on the elderly, and the results were not good for the aged. Some centers had stopped transplanting hepatitis B patients because the one-year survival rate was so low—the hepatitis always came back, often with more fury. Tom Starzl had chosen to use only baboon livers for hepatitis B patients, but Klintmalm still was offering human livers, with the caveat that the patient only got one shot. If the hepatitis destroyed the transplanted liver, that was it. No retransplant.

Now the question was whether the same standard should be applied to the elderly, since the numbers were even worse. "The elderly don't bounce back like a kid," someone noted. "There is no difference between age zero and age sixty,"

Levy offered. "From sixty to sixty-five, there is a drop. Then they drop off the cliff over sixty-five."

"When they are that sick and that old, they simply don't survive," another chimed in.

"We have some data now. We should learn from it," someone else said.

But the gastroenterologists continued to push, arguing that the surgeons were trying to change the rules in the middle of the game. They didn't know about this data. Let's talk about incorporating it into our rules in the future. Are you saying we should not look at anyone over sixty-five? Or just the sick ones? Regardless, this man is in the hospital, already on the fourteenth floor under the assumption that he would be up for a transplant shortly, and, being in the hospital, would take priority on the waiting list. Now this wrench gets thrown into the proceedings. Not fair. Not fair to him. Why shouldn't he get a chance?

Klintmalm had heard enough. "Look," he said sternly, "he can die after $150,000, or we can send him home to die."

The words hung heavily in the room. "He can die after $150,000." Is that what it boiled down to? No one wanted that. But no one wanted to send him home to die. Was there no chance? The gastroenterology staff just wanted the guy to have his chance. Who was going to explain to his family that they weren't even going to try to save his life? How could the surgeons make them out to be the bad guys?

A compromise was struck. What if they accepted him as a "status seven"—inactive—meaning that he was on the list, but too sick to be actively considered for a transplant? If he improved, got well enough for the transplant, then he would be activated, and would have already begun accumulating time on the list. If he got well enough to walk out of the hospital, not just be wheeled out in a chair but walk on his own legs by himself, then they would transplant him. That was easier to explain to the family. There would still be hope. If Roy Clover

■

could get home, he would get a chance to live on. But the compromise was far from popular.

"He may never get well enough to go home," one of the gastroenterology fellows protested.

"That's the point," Klintmalm shot back.

Ten days later, Roy Clover died, having never left the hospital.

Three weeks later, the selection committee accepted a seventy-year-old woman who, while not nearly as sick as Roy Clover, had trouble tolerating a simple nonsurgical procedure. If she had trouble with that, how could she make it through a liver transplant? At the same meeting, the committee voted in a sixty-six-year-old severely malnourished recovering alcoholic who had trouble with his veins and heart. "If you take the seventy-year-old, then you've got to take him," Bob Goldstein said.

And they did.

"I think we have to start making tougher choices," Goldstein said after the meeting. "It's getting easier for me to do, because of the shortage and because of the cost. Look at this *USA Today* story: 'Is Liver Transplantation Worth the Cost?' As the members of the committee get older and near retirement age, seventy doesn't look so old anymore. You could take someone seventy and give them ten years sitting on the porch in a rocking chair, ten years they earned and looked forward to. But we're going to have to begin making tougher choices."

For years the question had always been, can we give someone a new liver? Now surgeons could give just about anyone a new liver, and the question had become, should we give that person a new liver? It is a question that somebody will have to decide, society, government, someone. But for now, the decision is left to the doctors. The waiting lists grow longer and longer: Baylor was averaging three transplants a week, and six new patients before the selection committee each week. That kind of math will never add up. Where will the breaking point be? Will government have to set an age cutoff, as other countries have done? Will Americans accept being told that Mom, at age sixty-five, is too old for a liver transplant that might save her life and give her another five years with her grandchildren, maybe ten? Just how old is too old? Starzl's team in Pittsburgh did a transplant on a seventy-eight-year-old patient.

For now the policy decisions are left to the selection committee, and for the most part, they are left unmade. Each case gets a decision, but deciding anything case-by-case can result in some arbitrary-looking comparisons. Concerned that its policies were not firm enough, the group, over the course of 1993, took steps to tighten criteria and take some of the variability, even fickleness, out of the selection process. They studied the financial hurdles imposed on patients to make sure they were fair, and right. They moved to impose stricter standards on alcoholics: Six months of proven sobriety, with no exceptions. "Now it's a lot more consistent," Goldstein said. The committee examined and re-examined the age questions, working for more consistency in standards. And naturally, as the organ shortage grew worse and the waiting list grew longer, they became tougher gatekeepers forced to say "no" by the crisis of transplantation.

Yet, the reality is that the decisions can indeed seem inconsistent. One time the committee accepted one drug-and-alcohol user and rejected another. The differences boiled down to a question of one being liked, the other not. "Does he deserve a liver?" someone asked. The choices came down to who was most impressive in an interview with one of the committee members before the meeting, or who told a better story, or who looked more deserving of a chance at a miracle.

Timing can be a most difficult choice. No one wants a liver transplant before he absolutely has to have it. Yet no one wants to wait too long, wait until it is possibly too late, or at least until his chances of survival are diminished by the severity of his illness. There can be other factors. One man was a

■

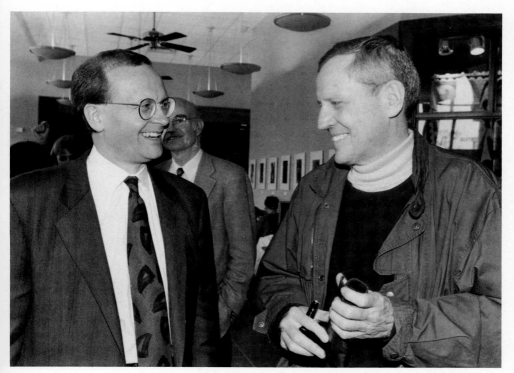

Goran Klintmalm (*left*) talks with Tom Starzl.

(Alison Victoria)

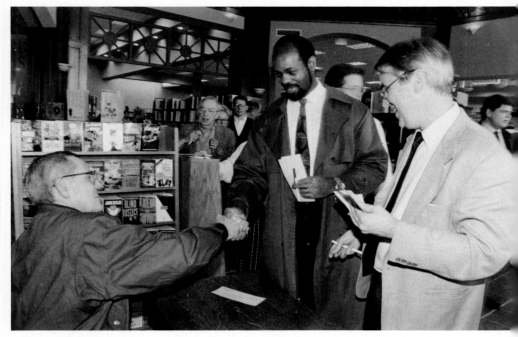

Dale Distant and Bo Husberg shake hands with Tom Starzl
at a book-signing for *The Puzzle People*. (*Alison Victoria*)

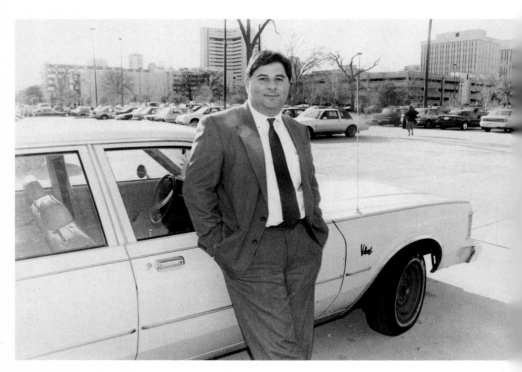

Marlon Levy with his 1979 Volare. (*Alison Victoria*)

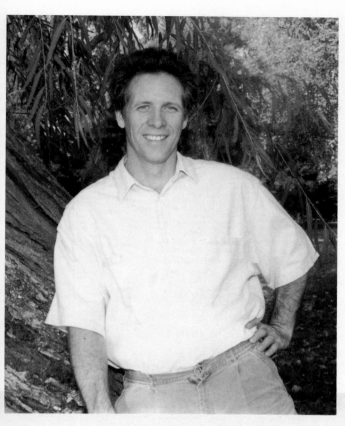

Bob Goldstein
(Alison Victoria)

Transplant coordinators
(left to right)
Sharon Anderson,
Pam Fertig,
Donna Morrissey,
and Sharon Carlen.
The four
are on the roof
of the Baylor University
Medical Center with
the skyline of Dallas
in the background.
(Alison Victoria)

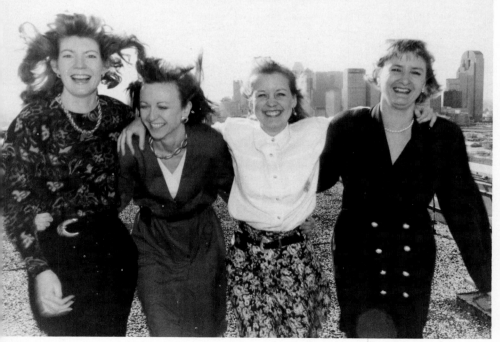

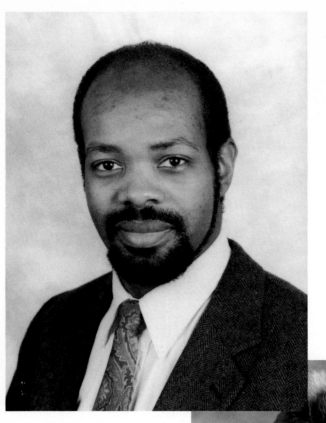

Dr. Dale Distant
*(Baylor University
Medical Center)*

Dr. Lars Backman
*(Baylor University
Medical Center)*

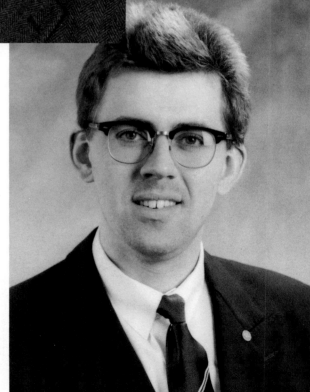

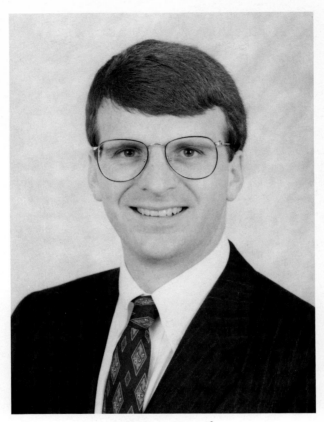

Dr. Tom Renard
(*Baylor University Medical Center*)

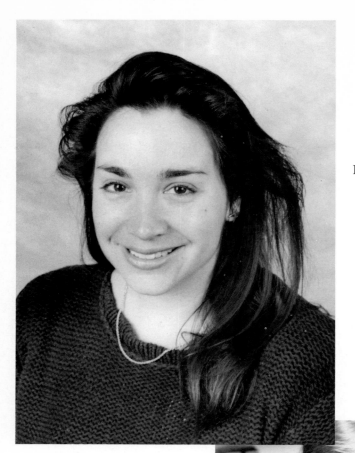

Dr. Caren Eisenstein
*(Baylor University
Medical Center)*

Caren Eisenstein
operates on a pig.
(Alison Victoria)

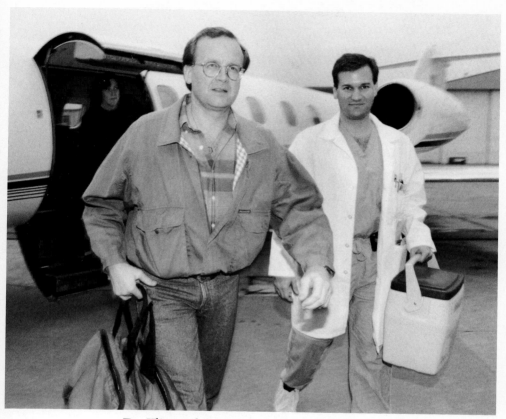
Dr. Klintmalm on a donor run. (*Alison Victoria*)

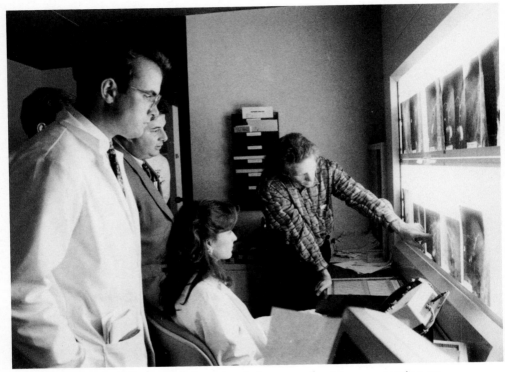

Bob Goldstein and the rest of the transplant team examine an
X-ray in the radiology department. (*Alison Victoria*)

Goran Klintmalm (*opposite*) at work with his loupes on.
(*Alison Victoria*)

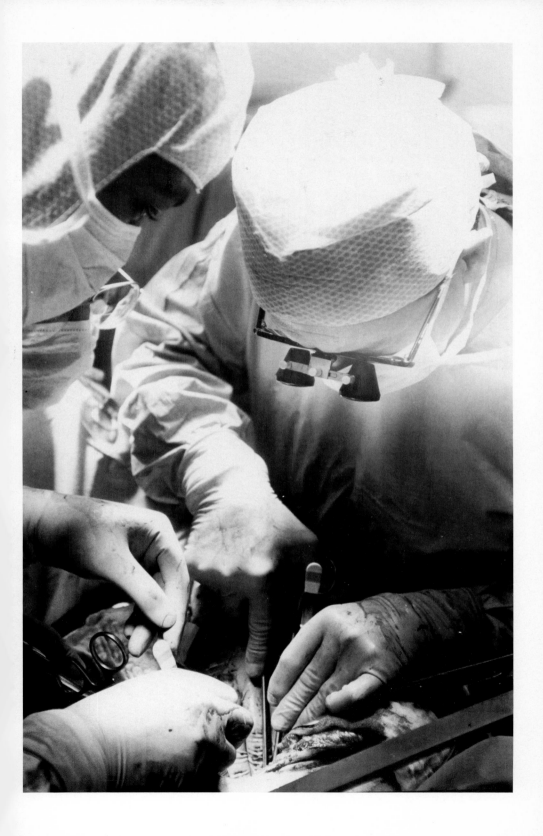

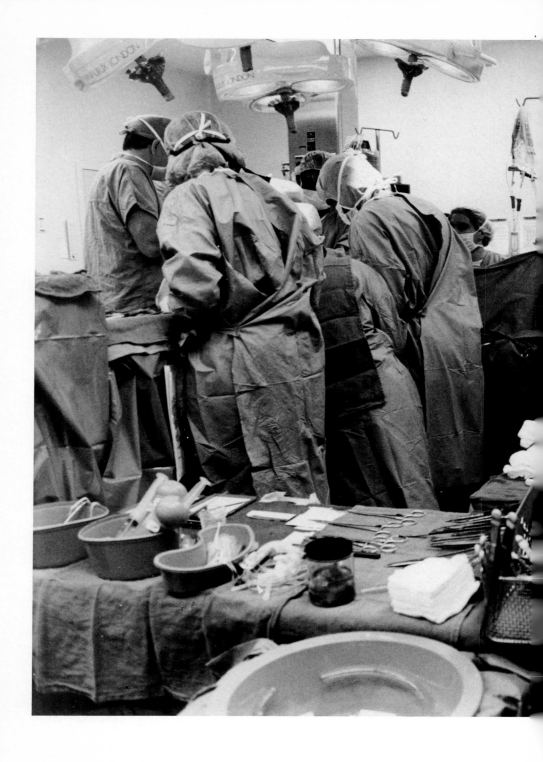

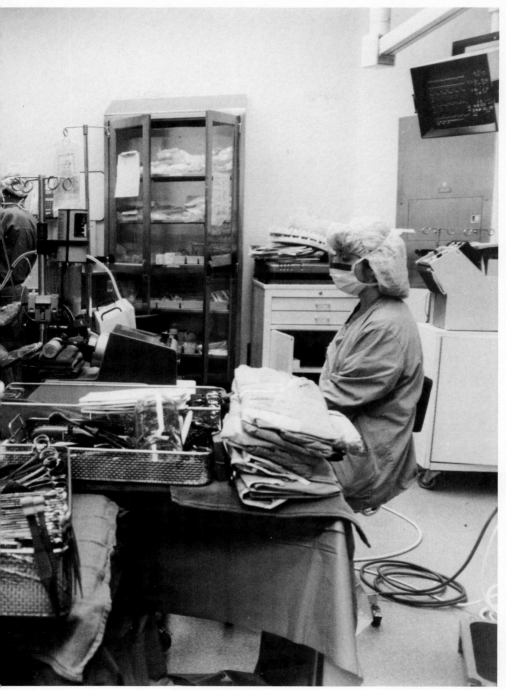

The scene in O.R. 4 at Baylor (Scott McCartney is at far left observing Mel Berg's surgery.) *(Alison Victoria)*

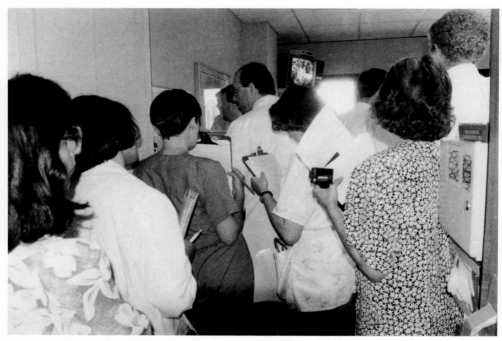

The transplant team crowds into a patient's room on rounds.
(Alison Victoria)

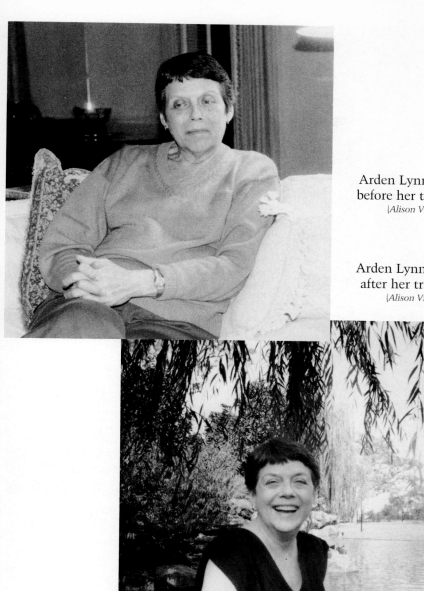

Arden Lynn at home
before her transplant.
(*Alison Victoria*)

Arden Lynn at Baylor
after her transplant.
(*Alison Victoria*)

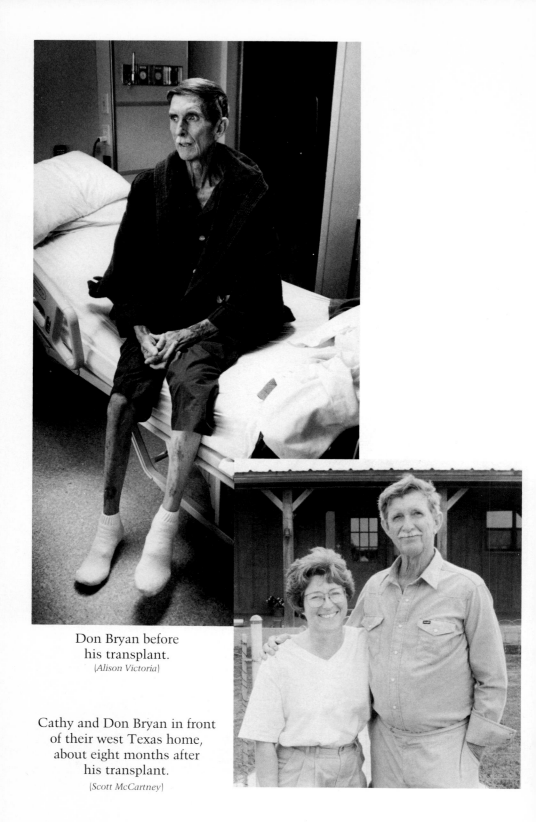

Don Bryan before
his transplant.
(Alison Victoria)

Cathy and Don Bryan in front
of their west Texas home,
about eight months after
his transplant.

(Scott McCartney)

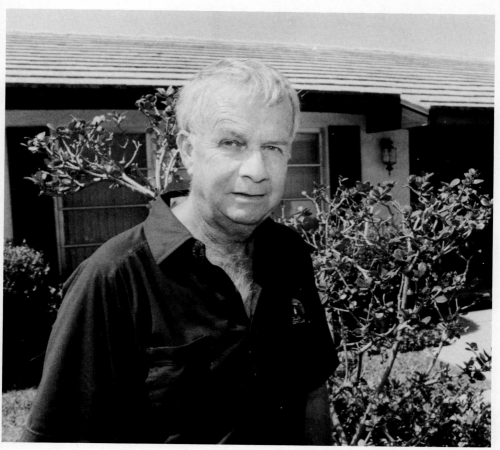

Mel Berg at his home in Jupiter, Florida, nine months after his transplant.
(Scott McCartney)

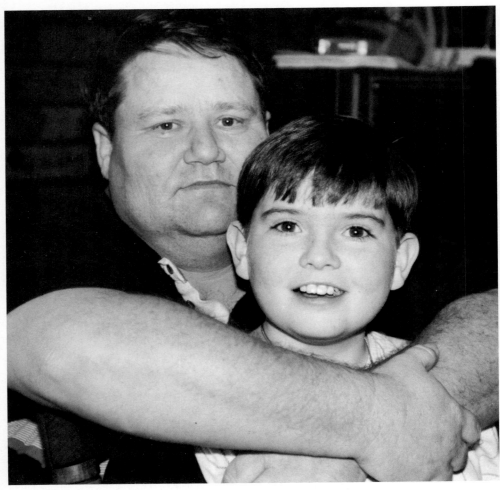

Randy Roady with his son, Heath.
(*Scott McCartney*)

bank vice president who was going downhill fast but probably was not yet sick enough for a new liver. Yet his bank had just been seized by the Federal Deposit Insurance Corporation the Friday before his Monday morning transplant evaluation appointment. His medical insurance would continue during the transition period, when the bank was operated by federal agents. But then what? Would he be out of a job or in a job with insurance that would not cover a transplant? He'd better get on this list now! The medical factors were overruled by the FDIC.

Two weeks before Christmas 1992, the committee accepted an even older seventy-year-old-woman who would turn seventy-one on the waiting list. She was a "young seventy" physiologically, and she expects to live to be ninety. "Medically, she was OK to accept," Dale Distant said after the meeting. "But morally, socially? That's another question. I don't know how to answer that one."

The same questions came up routinely in selection committee meetings. The same tough choices agonized over, with little final resolve. One week the committee accepted a sixty-seven-year-old with a stipulation that if he ended up in the intensive care unit while on the waiting list, he would not be a candidate, even though those that end up in the ICU usually move to the top of the list rather than get bumped off of it. Another time, a sixty-five-year old woman with poor kidney function was turned down—not in good-enough shape. What she really needed was a liver and a kidney, but she was a Medicare patient, and Medicare at the time refused to pay for transplanting more than one organ, so there was no point in considering that. She was turned down without a fight.

There are moments of levity in the selection committee, tension breakers needed almost as much here to ease the seriousness as in the intensive care unit. Everyone remembers the day that a patient with an alcoholic's cirrhosis of the liver was presented. Nobody liked the guy; there was just something raunchy about him. He needed a heart evaluation because he had been kicked in the chest violently by a mule, causing some damage. That brought chuckles. Then the committee turned to the social worker who had evaluated him, including an interview with his wife. Seems his wife found him so despicable that she had kicked him out of the house, and for a year and a half, he had been banished to living in the barn.

"The mule apparently didn't like him much better," someone remarked to uproarious laughter.

Then there was the day the committee was wrestling with the case of a young woman crazy about her pets. She was actually balking at going on the list for a liver transplant because pets were not allowed at Twice Blessed House, the apartment complex Baylor bought to house waiting and recovering transplant patients. In fact, pets are discouraged because they can carry diseases that could be disastrous for an immunosuppressed transplant patient. So fond of her animals was she that she was actually considering skipping the transplant altogether. The problem became a major discussion in the selection committee, raising the question of whether she really understood her plight, and whether she could make rational decisions about her medical care.

Dan Polter, usually silent during discussion until it comes time to vote, suddenly spoke.

"I guess," Polter said quietly, head pointed down into the papers before him, casting silence over the room, "she'll not want a baboon liver."

Hysteria.

Hard as the age questions may be, the toughest choices often arise when alcoholics come before the selection committee.

It used to be that only two or three percent of the patients receiving liver transplants were recovering alcoholics who had destroyed their "native livers" through drinking. But in 1990, Medicare began paying for transplants for alcoholics, and other insurance agencies fell in line. Now, nearly one-

■

quarter of the people getting new livers are alcoholics. The treatment of that disease has gained more and more acceptance by society. Alcoholism is viewed more and more as a disease, possibly even with a genetic link, and research shows that alcoholic cirrhosis is also likely to be the result of a physical defect in the liver—a trigger, such as an enzyme deficiency or an inherited liver disease—in addition to the drinking itself. And treatment of the effects of the disease is also gaining acceptance.

It remains controversial, however. Families agreeing to donate organs sometimes ask if the liver is going to a drunk. Doctors even grumble at times about "self-abusers." Including alcoholics has helped to lengthen the waiting lists; there is no penalty or provision for lower priority on the list. How can someone with a massive bout of hepatitis die because someone who drank too much took the only liver that might have saved his life?

"Should alcoholics get a liver on a lower priority? We debated that at length," Goldstein said. "We feel the answer is "no." They have a disease, like any other transplant patient. They should get a liver on medical requirements alone."

At Baylor, alcoholics do get more rigorous screening and must meet more requirements after the transplant. They must prove sobriety for six months by attending Alcoholics Anonymous or another accredited program. They must sign a contract pledging sobriety and recognizing that if they don't stay sober after the surgery, then the Baylor team will terminate care and the transplant patient will be on his own. The alcoholics, designated by a "Laennec's cirrhosis" diagnosis, are subject to random drug and alcoholic screening, including blood tests.

What transplant surgeons have found is that for alcoholics, past performance does not predict future drinking behavior. At Baylor, only thirteen percent of the alcoholics

■

transplanted have gone back to drinking. Survival from the surgery itself is as good as with the rest of the patients.

"Our committee tries to do the best we can to select people who will stay in rehabilitation," Goldstein assured a conference of organ bank workers meeting in Dallas, people charged with the duty of asking grieving families to consider donating organs. "Morally or medically, there is no good reason to preclude patients with alcoholic cirrhosis from fair consideration for liver transplantation."

But beyond all the testing and rules inevitably come the fuzzy areas. Whether someone has stopped drinking is almost always a judgment call, and the social worker may have a different opinion from the psychiatrist, the surgeon may have heard a different story from the gastroenterologist. "He may still be drinking" can be the kiss of death for a candidate in the selection committee, even, "He's still in denial that he has a problem." But those determinations can be impossible to make with certainty.

One man was turned down because he was an alcoholic working as a bartender, with two brothers in prison. Even though he was on a state medical program for the poor, he was suspected of keeping himself supplied with marijuana. "Is he dealing drugs?" No one wanted any part of him, even though he had not been charged with any crime.

Another man was turned down as too "slippery," with too much history of alcohol abuse and IV drug use. "He's not an all-star candidate," someone remarked. "I'm only presenting him because I think everyone deserves a chance," another doctor said, before he was unanimously turned down. "We'd be glad to refer him to another transplant center," someone suggested. A woman was turned down because she was a homeless alcoholic with no support system, no way to care for herself after the transplant, let alone pay for it in the first place.

Recounting these anecdotes without the context of the dozens and dozens of routine cases the committee ably deals with can make it all seem far more arbitrary than it is. That's not fair to the professionals forced to make what are, by definition, arbitrary choices. They do it with skill, grace, and compassion. "We are trying *very* hard to make decisions on issues that are extraordinarily difficult," Klintmalm said. Yet it is the difficult choices that stand out, and that offer a broader window into understanding just how difficult the choices are to make. Fate can indeed turn on who is able to be present at a meeting, and who isn't. The committee is no different than any other body of humans—it's just that its members are forced to make choices most people will never have to confront.

It was that way for the case of the sixty-one-year-old alcoholic who had jumped ahead of Don Bryan for a liver. He had been a debatable candidate before a testy committee, too. If he became any sicker, his GI doctor insisted, he would become too sick to operate on. But he had not proved the required sobriety. He had been a drinker for forty years and a heavy smoker. After he was told he had liver disease and needed to quit drinking immediately, he continued drinking for four years. He denied that the drinking affected his work; his wife whispered to a social worker in the hallway that he was only able to work half a day. It was a classic case: denial, continued abuse, all kinds of psychosocial factors in the family situation. The man couldn't get out of bed, but unlike Roy Clover, he was voted onto the active waiting list. (His case came up before standards on alcoholics were tightened.) Soon after the vote, he was moved to the intensive care unit, where he gained even greater priority on the waiting list.

After he received a new liver that weekend, the tension spilled over into the next committee meeting. Bo Husberg, the surgeon who had evaluated him, had not been present the week before because he was in surgery. He had expressed numerous reservations in his evaluation, but on the sheet presented to the committee, Husberg's comment was listed as simply "probably an acceptable candidate." His opinion had been miscast,

■

145

Husberg complained. The sheet should have been more elaborate. The guy had been railroaded through the committee.

The patient's gastroenterologist stormed out of the meeting, glaring at Husberg.

The game of picking and choosing never was much fun anyway.

CHAPTER 9
THE CHANCE FOR RANDY

Davis, Oklahoma, is home to 2,500 people, one stoplight, and a volunteer fire department. A haircut costs $5 at Royce Jones's barber shop, the kind straight out of Mayberry R.F.D. with the rack of tattered, ten-year-old magazines and a couple of deer heads mounted on the walls. It is the kind of town where everybody knows everybody, and everybody knows everybody's business. Davis lies fifty miles over the Texas border, near a popular recreation wilderness but not really close to much of anything, caught about halfway between *The Grapes of Wrath* and Norman Rockwell. Its rugged people struggle to make ends meet, dealing with the declining rural economy, declining business at the rock quarry that had employed a couple of generations, declining farm economy, declining downtown (blame it on the Wal-Mart), and declining population as kids grow up and move off to Dallas and Houston and Kansas City and Chicago. Still, it's as solid as America gets. Hardly anybody ever misses church in Davis, Oklahoma.

Randy Roady wears his red "Davis Wolves" cap with pride. Born and raised in Davis, Roady makes his family's ends meet with a host of jobs. He works in Davis's funeral home, he's second in command at the fire department, where he's helped out for fifteen years, and he's sexton of the town cemetery. He's been on the police department, worked in the grocery store. He's known all over town, a practical-joking, fun-loving, soft-spoken teddy bear with a kind heart from a big family. His wife, Cynthy, is a supervisor in a nearby state institution for the mentally retarded. They have three children, ages fourteen, ten, and seven, two girls, with a boy in the middle.

Never sick in his life, the beefy Roady began having nosebleeds in January 1992. And it took forever for the bleeding to stop. "I told him he's not going to die and leave me with three kids. He's going to go to the doctor," Cynthy said.

Severe fatigue set in. A seventy-five-year-old coworker was running circles around Roady at the funeral home. "There's something odd about this," Roady remembered thinking. When he began bleeding from his rectum, stubborn Randy Roady finally went to a doctor in Oklahoma City, who promptly told him he had cancer, then ruled that out, then told him it must be his liver, or maybe his spleen, the organ that holds reserve blood and lies across the abdomen on the left side of the body. Doctors decided to go in to remove Roady's spleen, but when they got into his belly they found a grossly diseased liver—so sick it would have shut down completely if they had removed the spleen. The surgeon biopsied his liver—stuck a hollow needle in to remove a tiny core for laboratory tests—and the organ turned into a fountain of blood. After sewing that up, stopping the bleeding, and closing Roady's belly, the Oklahoma City doctors suggested Roady needed a new liver.

"Oklahoma City had just started its program [at Memorial Hospital], and they had done only five livers. I heard the first four died, and I didn't like it. My insurance company wouldn't pay for Oklahoma City anyway. And my doctor hinted that I should go to Baylor," Roady said.

Randy and Cynthy Roady made the two-hour drive to Dallas from Davis in June for a week-long ordeal at Baylor. They innocently call it "evaluation," but it is much more. To some, it can be the most grueling and nerve-wracking experience of the entire transplant ordeal. Every vital inch of the body

■

is checked. Are the kidneys strong enough to withstand the toxic medication a transplant requires? Is the heart strong enough? The lungs? The stomach? The mind? . . . Is the patient "psychosocially" strong enough? Is there family support? History of alcoholism? Smoking? The causes of the liver disease are probed. What are the risk factors for hepatitis? Any tattoos? Intravenous drug use? Traveled in Asia or elsewhere abroad? Ever been with a prostitute? What kind of patient will you be? Is there any track record of not following doctors orders?

All week, different specialists probe and question, each one probably capable of blackballing the patient when the time comes for review in the selection committee the following Wednesday. For Randy and most other patients, suddenly the focus of fear is not the disease but the committee that must accept them into the miracle machine. Did the social worker like me? What did the surgeon mean by that question? Why did they send me to a cancer specialist?

"I kept wondering, 'Why me?' " Roady said. "I guess everyone asks that question."

Roady's diseased liver—cirrhosis—appeared to be the work of a virus, probably some unknown form of hepatitis. Because he worked in the funeral home embalming bodies and handling blood, Roady was at high risk for hepatitis, but he tested negatively for all three testable strains, although there was some indication that he had been exposed to hepatitis B and hepatitis C but had not contracted the diseases. Today, doctors have identified hepatitis A, B, C, D, and E. Hepatitis F, and more, are on the way. And there are tests now for hepatitis A, B, and C. But liver specialists know there are a host of hepatitis viruses out there not yet identified, and certainly not yet testable. The test for hepatitis C is only a few years old. Until there was a test, the virus existed in some stored units of blood, and many people who got hepatitis C got it from simple transfusions during routine surgery.

■

Finding no other reason for Roady's damaged liver, he was labeled "cryptogenic cirrhosis"—diseased, but they don't know why.

"I really couldn't say where I got it," Randy said.

Klintmalm evaluated Roady and declared him an "appropriate patient for transplant. The question of his hepatitis is unclear and would need some further investigation before final treatment protocols are established."

The week following his evaluation, Roady was told he had been accepted by the committee and was offered a spot on Baylor's waiting list. All he had to do was obtain his insurance company's agreement to cover the cost, get a local beeper in Oklahoma, and sit tight—if he wanted to do it.

"For me, it was a tough decision. I've never seen numbers like $150,000. Why spend that much money for me? Why go through all that when you might not live anyway? It still seems like a dream. I can't see it happening, and can't believe I'm sick enough to do something like that."

But Klintmalm had told Roady he had only three to six months to live with the liver he had now. That made for a pretty convincing argument.

"I went on the list because I want to live. I'm not scared about the surgery, not scared about the recovery after it. What's scary is, how long do I have after I'm out of here? People here are happy with five or ten years. I'm thirty-eight. Five or ten years is not enough. Will I live to be fifty-eight? Sixty-eight? They don't know."

While on the waiting list, Cynthy and Randy began trying to explain the uncertain future to their three children, telling each that Daddy might die.

"Even my little girl understands what's going on. She's been real loving. She stops and kisses me, 'I love you Daddy.' But she's had bad dreams. In the middle of the night she started talking about heaven and woke up once grabbing her sides and screaming, 'No Daddy! No Daddy!' "

■

His son, Heath, handled it differently. Almost insepa-
rable from his father for the past few years and terribly proud of
Randy, Heath suddenly began rejecting him, pushing him away
out of anger and fear. "I hate you!" he shouted one day and ran
out the door. The pain of dealing with an anguished son was
almost worse than his own illness. Nothing hurt Randy more
than to see Heath casting him away. It wasn't until much later
that he realized Heath was simply scared.

Money was another part of the crisis. Blue Cross/Blue
Shield of Oklahoma, Roady's insurance through the funeral
home, would pay only a portion of the cost of the transplant—
the bulk, but no more than eighty percent. That left at least
$30,000, and probably much more, Roady would have to pay.
And the insurance would not cover the organ bank's cost of getting the liver, another $19,000. Nothing would cover lost
income and steep living expenses away from home in Dallas.

Word spread through Davis that Randy Roady was sick,
very sick, and had gone off to Dallas for a liver transplant. Soon
the fund-raisers began, spearheaded by his friends at the fire
department. There were Randy Roady Auctions, Randy Roady
Garage Sales, a Randy Roady Carnival, a Randy Roady Softball
Tournament, a Randy Roady Raffle. Some of the mentally
retarded residents of the institution made a quilt to be auc-
tioned. Donor cards were distributed around town and signed
as the community became more aware of the organ shortage.
On the front page of the weekly *Davis News*, the status of
Randy Roady's benefits was chronicled. If the Roadys went out
to eat, someone almost always paid the check for them. At the
utility company, strangers in line to pay bills stepped forward
and covered Roady's electricity bill. A beeper company donated
the beeper when it learned Randy was a transplant patient.
Coworkers of Cynthy's bought up raffle tickets. "I feel so
guilty," she said. "Single parents making less money than me
and here they are helping me."

In six months, Davis, Oklahoma, town of 2,500, had

■

raised $25,000 for a dying favorite son. "Davis is the kind of town where we don't know any better. We just get the job done. We always believe we can do it," says Royce Jones, the barber.

As exciting as the town charity was, it was debilitating to Randy, who never before had to ask for a handout. As his skin turned darker and darker shades of mustard brown, friends began looking at him a little strangely, acting as if they saw a ghost. Then the question kept popping up: When are they going to get that liver for you? Haven't they got a liver for you yet? When? When? When?

The long wait had begun. It took Blue Cross six weeks to clear Roady financially, meaning he wasn't actually put on Baylor's waiting list until six weeks after the selection committee had accepted him. Unable to work more than a few hours here and there, Roady sank lower and lower, physically and emotionally. As his body deteriorated, he worried more and more that he would be too sick to get a transplant, or too sick to survive. Why was it taking so long? Why couldn't they get him a liver? Had they forgotten about him? He was embarrassed to go to the Friday night football games. "Hey Randy," a friend would bark innocently, "Why haven't they got a liver for you yet?"

"It's like walking through hell with gasoline on your hands," he said during the wait. "It's all I know so far, but it's really hard. I jump when the phone rings and listen in real closely. And the phone rings a lot with a fourteen-year-old in your house."

Dealing with his own family became tougher and tougher too. He became afraid to discipline his children, fearing that the last thing they might remember about Daddy was a grouchy punishment. "I tried to be tough with them. They'd ask for eight cookies, and I'd say, 'No. You can have seven.' " He felt like he had become a burden, and he hated it.

"I started thinking, This is crazy, me getting a liver transplant. It's not worth the money, it's not worth the hurt on everyone. It might not work anyway. Maybe I should just end it all now and save a lot of trouble."

When his thoughts of suicide crept in, Cynthy recognized trouble and whisked Randy back to Baylor, where he was admitted to a psychiatric unit for two weeks and treated for deep depression. With those waiting on the transplant list, depression is about as common as fluid retention.

Bobby Murray, the Capitol police officer from Washington, visited Roady in the psychiatric unit regularly, and the two became joke-around friends. Roady began attending the regular Wednesday support group meetings for transplant patients—one for those being evaluated, and one for those already transplanted. Because he was on the list, Roady could attend both. After he returned to Davis, he continued to commute to the support group each week. There he found people who understood what he was going through. Most weeks Randy sat there silently in the meetings, absorbing. It was the one place he did not feel out of place, the one place where there was both hope and reality. The support group was something to look forward to each week, an excuse to show his face around Baylor and remind them he was waiting, a chance to hear war stories from those who had been through it. The support group, in a sense, saved his life by keeping him going.

In August, a sixteen-year-old girl Randy had known for years was killed in a car accident just outside town. She had signed the back of her driver's license to be an organ donor, and her family made a special request in their moment of ultimate grief: They wanted her liver to go to Randy Roady. "I don't know if I could have thought of something like that at a time like that," Cynthy said later. "It's one heck of a town we live in."

The Oklahoma organ bank contacted Baylor and found that the liver was the wrong blood type for Randy, and was too small for his girth. But it ended up at Baylor anyway, transplanted into a woman who recovered fully and returned to her home and family far healthier than before.

■

And the wait continued for Randy, who helped work the girl's funeral.

After sixteen weeks on the list, Randy Roady was staggering, sliding, sleeping all the time and yet nervous and anxious as a death-row inmate on appeal. Doctors had told him he was first on the list—but that was two weeks ago, and he soon learned that didn't mean much. Cynthy pondered unpacking both suitcases and running the car out of gas just to prompt the phone call to come when they were least prepared. Randy had to go to his local doctor Friday, throwing up blood. "People stared at me. I wanted to say, 'I'm alive,' " Randy said.

On Sunday night, October 26, the Roady family was preparing to go to church when the phone rang with the news that a liver had been found that was the right size and blood type for Randy. Randy promised Donna Morrissey that they would be there within three hours, then turned to his sister and said, "This is it." Soon the news was broadcast over the police radio, the fire radio, even Channel 7 television. There was a liver for Randy Roady. Finally! Seventeen weeks after he got on the list, twenty-three weeks after he had been evaluated and told the wait might be a month, maybe two.

Police cars and fire trucks lined up at the Roady home to escort the patient out to the interstate, sirens and lights on. The entourage got as far as the Santa Fe railroad tracks only to be blocked by a stopped train. Soon the police chief was threatening to jail everyone aboard if they didn't move their train from that intersection. Another thirty-minute delay.

Randy talked about the surgery on the way down to Dallas, scared at what was about to happen to him. He arrived at Baylor with his entire extended family, parents, brothers, sisters, kids, spouses—eighteen in all. Dale Distant began the prepping, ordering an electrocardiogram, a chest X ray, everything down to suppositories and enemas. The vampire showed up with the twenty-five empty blood-sample tubes to be filled. Distant took Roady's history.

■

"There are no guarantees, but we help most people," he told Randy, compassion evident with each word. "I'm available all night for other questions."

A slew of consent forms had to be signed, allowing an AIDS test, releasing the donor family from any liability. There was one that would place Randy into a study of a new immuno-suppressant drug, FK 506. FK 506 was more powerful than cyclosporine and initially had been touted as the magic miracle pill all had been awaiting. It didn't turn out quite that good, but it did seem to work slightly better than cyclosporine. Tom Starzl had helped Baylor become one of only a few sites testing the drug before approval from the Food and Drug Administration, and now a study was under way to determine the optimal doses of FK to give. Roady was hesitant.

"We think it's a good drug," Distant said. "It's more powerful, and we've had good results with it. But it's totally up to you."

Roady signed up.

"It's not as scary now," he said as nurses and technicians continued the preparations. "I'm just wondering what they're going to do next and focusing on what it will be like afterwards. I love to go to Galveston on vacation, and so I'm thinking about that. Walking on the beach in the morning. Going crabbing at night with flashlights. And I got with my oldest sister and friend and told them all what to do if I don't make it, but I'm going to make it.

"One other question," Randy said to Distant who had returned to the room to collect the forms. "You know where this liver is coming from?"

"It's either Corpus Christi or Galveston. They're going to both places tonight," he said.

"A Texas liver for an Oklahoma boy?!" Randy exclaimed. "I'm sure it's Galveston. I love Galveston."

The Galveston liver had almost been ruled unacceptable. On the back table, a heart surgeon flown in to harvest discovered some vegetation growth on his valves—possibly the result of intravenous drug use. Vegetation can lead to bacterial infection, and one big no-no in transplanting is putting an infected organ into a recipient who, because the immune system is suppressed, may be unable to fight off the infection.

"It [finding the growth] was a total surprise," Klintmalm said later.

Caren Eisenstein, who had flown to Galveston with Klintmalm for the retrieval, kept asking what he was going to do, and he was obviously not sure what to do. "We have to think about this," Klintmalm kept saying. With kidneys, if the transplant is lost to infection the patient can always just go back to dialysis. But with a liver, the result might be death. Even in transplanting, the physician's credo is "First, do no harm." But these days, with the list never ending and patients dying while waiting for livers, the choices are not as simple as catchy credos chiseled in marble. "Doing harm" might mean throwing away a liver that might save someone's life. Or "doing harm" might mean transplanting a horribly deadly infection. There is no way to teach easy answers to the choices transplant surgeons face now.

Klintmalm, operating on just six hours sleep in two nights, consulted on the phone with his team back in Dallas. Finding no evidence of infection in the liver, he decided to use it, but the recipient had to agree to a long course of antibiotics just to make sure any infection would be killed. He called back to Dallas, and Roady was informed of the problem.

"If you don't want it, we will use it on someone," Distant had told him.

"I'll take it," Randy replied.

The heart was not used, the pancreas was not used, but the kidneys were. The heart was taken back to Dallas for further pathology tests, an effort to protect Randy by probing further the cause and extent of the vegetation. It was another case

■

of Klintmalm, driven by the waiting list and his own confidence, stretching the envelope.

By midnight, the Roady children were beyond scared and into bleary-eyed exhausted. A chaplain was on his way in for last-minute comforting and praying. "You all go kiss your daddy, then we're going to go lie down," Cynthy said.

At 4:30 A.M., Randy Roady was wheeled out of the room on fourteen and taken down to the second-floor operating suite. Cynthy followed for as long as she was allowed. They exchanged "I love you"s, then Cynthy kissed Randy and said "See ya later." Then he was gone, whisked off into the world of new-frontier medicine. Cynthy cried, went downstairs, and stood in front of the hospital, chain-smoking half a pack of cigarettes. "I have no doubt at all that I'll see him later. No doubt at all."

A little after 5 A.M., Dale Distant, himself up most of the night, began opening Randy Roady, an Oklahoma boy about to get his Galveston liver. It had come from a twenty-one-year-old troubled youth who had been playing Russian roulette with his friends. "I don't know if that means he won or lost," said Eisenstein. After Galveston, she and Klintmalm had flown on to Corpus Christi for another liver, which Bo Husberg would transplant following Roady's surgery. At the moment, Husberg was doing a kidney transplant; Marlon Levy was working with Distant, teaching and supervising.

Roady proved to be a difficult case in the operating room, tiring to the surgeons because he was beefy, tricky technically because he bled a great deal. Still, the banter was lively in O.R. 4 as the sun came up, and the surgeons were busy. They're always happier when busy. Tom Renard stuck his head in to announce that it was Marlon's birthday, and a chorus of "Happy Birthday" went up. Bob Goldstein phoned in from home, calling to say goodbye to Marlon as he headed off on a three-week vacation to climb Mount Everest. "Thanks

Bob, have a good time," Marlon yelled at the receiver sarcastically.

"Call me if you need me," Goldstein chuckled back, heading off to Nepal—without his beeper.

The joking disappeared as Levy called for Roady's new liver. Blood flow through the bypass was falling, an anesthesiologist was squeezing new blood into Roady by hand, and Distant, his feet in a pool of blood that had run over the side of Randy's gut, was sucking fresh blood from the abdomen as fast as he could with the Cell Saver.

"Flow down to one liter," the bypass machine technician called out.

"Flow is point six."

"We're coming off bypass," Levy responded.

As the portal vein was released and blood flowed, the donated liver slowly turned from a caramel-brown color to purple.

But the bleeding continued.

"Let's dig out the anastomosis," Levy suggested, hunting for the source of the bleeding.

"Stupid son of a bitch," he muttered in frustration.

"Bovie!" he called.

Not a word was spoken. Four heads and four light pods were aimed at Roady's abdomen, seven or eight hands in there at one time all looking for bleeding.

"On the artery, you think?" asked Levy, his gown now bloodied like a butcher's apron. "Can we make it cooler in here?!"

"Check the coag numbers," Levy said to the anesthesiologist, wondering about the status of Roady's ability to coagulate his blood, slow down the bleeding, and increase the volume of blood in his body.

"We're just offsetting," the anesthesiologist responded.

"And how's the coagulating?"

"Terrible."

■

"It could be surgical, we don't know."

Was there a wound or opening through which Roady was bleeding, or was he bleeding simply because his blood was unable to clot, as before the transplant, because it was so low on coagulating factors produced by the liver?

Marlon Levy threw his head back, toward the ceiling, stretching his neck to ease a tension that could almost be touched in the operating room.

"You're skimming," he said to Distant, who was sewing up Roady's hepatic artery. "You're skimming." Sewing the donor hepatic artery to Roady's proved especially difficult because they were different sizes. The donor's was about as wide as a pencil; Randy's as wide as a thumb. So Distant narrowed Roady's and then made the anastomosis.

"Artery's open," Levy announced.

By now, Roady had consumed eight units of blood from the blood bank, and seven units of his own recycled with the Cell Saver. He wasn't the worst bleeder they had seen—not even the worst of the week. Two days earlier a patient bled so much that Husberg had to summon Klintmalm from home. The patient consumed thirty units of blood—but even that was a far cry from the early days of liver transplants when the surgery could last twenty-four hours and drain a city's entire blood bank.

Randy Roady wasn't nearly that bad. But he was a bleeder.

"You're not happy?" Levy, sensing uncertainty under the surgical mask, said to Distant as he prepared to close Roady's chest by lacing him up.

"I'm just worried about the bleeding."

"There's nothing to do but close. Nothing you can do surgically. He's just coagulopathic, and his liver function will improve that."

On the fourteenth floor, Levy found a horde of red-hatted Davis Wolves, as if a new cult had descended on Baylor. "It went very well," he told the family. "We used fifteen units of blood, and there was a little more bleeding than usual. They're sewing him up now, and he'll be in ICU soon."

"How optimistic are you, doctor?" someone asked nervously.

"Reasonably optimistic."

Levy surveyed the dozen-plus family members in the hospital suite used for waiting families and began trying to identify and meet each one, shaking hands with political fervor. Like a circus car, the red caps kept coming. "You guys have the record," he said cheerfully. "We'll see you later."

The family formed a circle and prayed. Cynthy, who had had all of one hour of sleep, cried.

CHAPTER 10

THE NUMBERS GAME I

The transplant intensive care unit, 4 East, was like a battlefield, casualties lined up everywhere the eye fell. The unit had been full until Bobby Murray, who had befriended Randy Roady only to end up two beds away in the ICU, had died. Randy didn't know about his friend and role model Murray; Cynthy decided it would be better for his recovery not to hear about it for a week or two. Still, all around him was a hodgepodge of people trying to pull one over on the gods.

In one bed, Yolanda Contreras was having seizures, struggling to stay alive. She had not awakened from her surgery, which had been just four days ago, and, still in a coma, appeared to be close to vegetable status mentally. On top of that, she had turned bright yellow—jaundiced from poor liver functions. Her body was rejecting her liver, attacking the foreign matter transplanted inside her.

In another bed lay her surgical "twin," a Tulsa, Oklahoma, woman who had been transplanted while in a coma brought on by a massive attack of hepatitis. She had not come out of her coma either and appeared to have just as slim a chance of survival as Contreras.

As if those two did not provide enough agony, a woman named Nora Barnes, transplanted just ten days before, had returned to the ICU because of seizures. But there was no

■

apparent cause for the seizures and shaking. The surgeons thought it must be a brain or spinal problem, but the neurologists couldn't find anything wrong. The neurologists thought it must be a lung problem, but the pulmonary specialists could find nothing amiss and suggested heart trouble. The cardiologists found nothing and suggested pulmonary trouble. Everything was great, nothing was wrong, the specialists pledged—except Nora Barnes was circling the drain.

On the way into the unit on rounds, Goran Klintmalm was telling his team about the recent transplant. Husberg had summoned him back to Baylor, interrupting his business dinner before drinks or appetizers. When Klintmalm walked into O.R. 4 and surveyed the scene, he suggested to a visiting medical school student that this was the way they did all their transplants. "What is this?" she asked innocently of Husberg, pointing somewhere. "This," the usually mild-mannered Swede shouted, "IS A GODDAMNED MESS!"

Klintmalm howled at Husberg's outburst. "I was called in before my martini, and I got a Bloody Mary instead," he chuckled. The patient survived.

The team, nearing the end of an exhausting stretch of seven liver transplants, seven liver harvests, and two kidney transplants in just six days, was laughing heartily as it entered the ICU, confronted at the desk by a group of weary nurses puzzled at the laughter amid the carnage.

"Why are you laughing?" one nurse asked Klintmalm, exasperation dripping from her voice.

"Oh, if we can't have fun, what's the point," he exclaimed, chuckling all the way.

Laughter. It's like Valium for the transplant team's stress.

Next door to Randy, a career air force veteran was recovering nicely with the Corpus Christi liver that Klintmalm had retrieved the same night as Roady's Galveston liver. He was a

■

sign of normalcy amid the chaos. On this day, a patient doing well seemed like a rarity.

As the team moved to Randy's bedside, Dale Distant recounted the surgery. "This was a difficult hepatectomy," Distant said, "because he's fat."

Randy woke up as Klintmalm moved to his bedside. "Hi, time to get up," he yelled in his clearest Swinglish.

"Mr. Roady is doing well, although he may be difficult to wean from the ventilator," Distant said.

Because he had been a longtime smoker and had a big chest, Randy's lungs would be slow to recover from the surgery and for several days would require the assistance of a breathing machine. That meant no talking and nothing by mouth, not even ice chips to ease the throat. It also meant a constant choking feeling. Pain is part of the process because too much sedation slows recovery after transplant.

Cynthy told Randy she would stay all night in the ICU waiting room, rather than return to the apartment the family had been rented at Twice Blessed House, a thirty-four-unit apartment building Baylor runs for transplant patients.

"G-O" Randy wrote on her hand with a pen.

"No," she insisted. She would stay.

"P" Randy wrote.

"P? Do you need to pee?"

No, Randy shook.

"Pain? Are you in pain?"

He nodded yes, and then wrote "W" on the hand.

"Water?" Yes, he wanted water, but it was forbidden.

Then, Randy Roady, struggling to breathe after his belly had been sliced wide open and his insides rearranged, if not replaced, grabbed the pen to write one more thought.

"I L-O-V-E Y-O-U."

The visit was over.

In the Baylor ICU, families are allowed fifteen minutes

with the patient several times a day. Otherwise, they are relegated to a communal waiting room down the hall from the large, mechanical ICU doors. No children are allowed. The first night after surgery, Randy's ten-year-old son Heath begged his mother and the nurses to go see his father. They all said no. Children can heighten the risk of infection. It was too soon.

Heath Roady slammed his body into the wide doors, bawling, crying because he could not go see his father.

Twice a day Cynthy received updates from the doctors. Randy was doing well, they usually said, not breathing as much as they would like, however. Velton Smith, the air force veteran transplanted the same day as Randy, already had been transferred out of intensive care and up to the fourteenth floor, a sign of discouragement for the Roadys.

Still, how could they not be excited?

"I'm high," Cynthy said, bubbling. "The doctors have been *wonderful*. They describe everything, and they have been so friendly. I got to see Klintmalm himself yesterday. And the kids got to go in a bit and see Randy from a distance. He waved to them." In her eyes, the doctors who had given her husband a second chance were themselves gods.

Further lab results began coming back on Randy's donor, each bringing good news. Blood and urine cultures were negative, indicating the infection in the donor was very limited and the risk to Randy minimal. A biopsy of the new liver showed some degeneration but not anything beyond the normal damage caused during preservation of the liver. It looked as if in the case of this very tough call, Klintmalm had made the right choice.

With triumphant smiles, the Roady family returned to the support group two days after Randy's transplant to boast about their good fortune and thank the now-tight circle of friends who had supported Randy through the waiting. He was still in the ICU, but they took their excitement to the group any-

■

way. They told about how "sky-high" they were. They told about how Heath had cried outside the ICU door. They talked about how excited they were, and the group shared their wonder.

Then another transplant patient asked social worker Michelle Long how Bobby Murray was doing. "He died yesterday," she said. The group talked about the small percentage that do die, and they remembered Murray and his family, regulars themselves in the support group. No one is bulletproof but most do well, they all reassured themselves. It's hard to figure out why some do well and some do so poorly. Medicine can't predict. Who can? For transplant patients, the question always comes up: Why him, instead of you?

"Well, that happens sometimes," ten-year-old Heath Roady told the group, his enthusiasm for his father's chances seemingly undiminished.

Yet the days in the ICU waiting room began to drag on, and each one brought a little more worry for Cynthy Roady. Most patients were out of the ICU and up to the fourteenth floor in a day or two. Now Randy had been there four days, five days, six days. He still couldn't breathe for himself—there was too much fluid in his chest. Doctors drained twenty-five pounds of fluid from Randy one night, but it still was not enough. Each day she would ask when he might be moved out of the ICU and up to the fourteenth floor. Each day the answer was "maybe tomorrow." Each tomorrow the answer was the same. One lesson of Bobby Murray's death was on everyone's mind: The longer you stay in the ICU, the worse your chances are. No doubt about that. The roller coaster ride of highs and lows had begun. Cynthy Roady, who had visited with Bob Murray's wife to console her after his death, was sinking after the initial high of the transplant.

For the transplant team, Roady was a minor problem. There was still a full load of eight patients in the intensive care unit. Discussion had begun about removing Nora Barnes, the woman who had the mystery disease, from her life-support machine. Pulling the plug was the only option the doctors had left now. But a day before the plug was to be pulled, her heart gave out, and she died. The autopsy found nothing wrong, except that she was dead, less than two weeks after the transplant.

Another patient transplanted for cancer turned out, according to the pathology reports, to have cancer in her bile ducts as well as her liver, meaning her chances of survival were greatly diminished. The Contreras and Leonard "sisters" were both still in comas. Another patient transplanted in that same hectic six-day stretch was having seizures and talking irrationally. But in his stupor, he announced that he had been sexually molesting his daughter. On top of that, his bile duct was leaking. There was the sweet, tiny elderly woman who had suffered a stroke after senior fellow Lars Backman pulled her T-tube. And there was the most recent transplant, a patient who appeared to be rejecting his new liver immediately and, after just twenty-four hours, was relisted for another emergency transplant.

"Look at all the ventilators," one of the surgical residents remarked as the team walked into the ICU. "No need to air-condition this place."

It seemed never to end. Klintmalm tried mustering some humor, joking about sedating the doctors, kidding the fellows about the size of their biopsy specimens. But for the first time, it didn't seem to be helping much. The strain was showing.

In the X ray–viewing room, Goran Klintmalm punched up Randy Roady's daily chest X ray to see if the fluid in his chest was clearing.

"That looks better," he said proudly.

"That's not Roady," Lars Backman noted. "That's why it looks better."

When they switched to Randy's X ray, on the upper tier

■

of a two-tier viewing board, Klintmalm found that it actually did look a little bit better.

"Randy is still having trouble breathing," Klintmalm later told Cynthy Roady in the waiting room upstairs. "He's barely making it on his own. We'll keep him in the ICU at least until tomorrow, probably the next day."

Two patients in the room next door to Randy had now come and gone from the ICU. The week had twisted so slowly, so painfully, that it seemed like an eternity. As the team left, Cynthy had a tear in her eye. She grabbed the hand of Heath, who was suddenly growing up very quickly, and turned to leave, mother and son, hand in hand, holding on to each other for support.

The front page of the *Davis News* carried a bold headline: "Roady Has Successful Transplant Operation." For Davis, the news couldn't have been sweeter. After a grueling stint, Randy Roady was finally out of intensive care, sixty pounds lighter than before his transplant. For the first time in years, his wedding band fit on his finger. For the first time in years, he was beginning to feel better. And for the first time since the transplant more than a week ago, he could breathe pretty well on his own.

On the fourteenth floor, it was beginning to look as if Randy had turned the corner. An orange banner signed by most of Davis covered the window in his room; get-well cards were taped across another wall. Finally, for perhaps the first time in the six months or so that he had been coming to Baylor Medical Center, Randy Roady smiled.

As part of the routine, dye was injected into Randy's bile duct system through the T-tube in a test to X-ray how good flow was through the vessels. Randy's thumb-sized duct had been tightened to match the pencil-wide donor bile duct. Now, as Marlon Levy read the X rays, trouble appeared—the X rays showed an enlargement of the tissue-tube where the two ends were sewn together. The ballooning of the vessel might mean there was a blockage, meaning bile might not be able to get through the duct. It's something like a busy highway intersection at rush hour, and the danger is that the liver wouldn't empty all the bile it needs to.

"The conservative thing to do," Levy said to the team in the X ray–viewing room at the start of rounds, "is to take this man back to the O.R. and fix this."

In Randy's room, the patient was in good cheer, convinced all was well. Marlon Levy began quickly explaining the results of the T-tube test. He would clamp the T-tube drain and see how it went. If his liver function numbers keep improving, then there would be no problem. But if they worsened, there was a problem—a problem that might have to be fixed in the operating room. They would have to open him up and fix the bile duct connection.

As Levy left, Randy suddenly became teary-eyed. From the top of the roller coaster he had plunged to the bottom in a matter of seconds. From "I'm doing great" to "I'm going back to the operating room." What a blow. A nurse tried to calm him down, and soon word was relayed back to Levy that Randy Roady needed to see him again after rounds. It was all a shock. Could the doctor explain it some more?

"Dr. Levy came back last night and said it was not that big a deal. I wanted an explanation because they just turned around from the chart and said, 'OK, if the duct is not going to fix itself, we'll take you to surgery Friday.' I said, 'What?!' And they turned around and were gone."

"I'll do anything to avoid this surgery," he added the next day, anxiously awaiting the posting of his lab results—his numbers—on the wall chart in his room.

In transplanting, the numbers are everything—the thing the patients live by, the factor the doctors examine most closely. Believing that transplant patients have to take responsibility for and should be involved in decisions about their care, the daily lab results are publicly posted in each room before rounds. When the team enters the patient's room, all eyes go straight to the yard-long wall chart, which is hung on the wall opposite the bed. Patients can easily feel relegated to second-class status compared to that chart. It's as if the doctors ask the chart how it's doing before acknowledging there is a person in the room. It can be a source of aggravation for patients when the team members come in, immediately turn their backs and mumble among themselves as they pore over the numbers produced by blood tests. Sometimes, there can be long, hushed discussions, then a turn toward the patient and a simple "Everything is fine. See you tomorrow."

The numbers are the result of blood tests drawn at five or six o'clock in the morning. After lunch, a secretary from Klintmalm's office makes her own rounds on the floor, posting numbers in pencil on the wall charts. Her visit is often more welcome, or more dreaded, than those of the doctors. She is the one who brings good news or bad, and even before the transplant team arrives a couple of hours later, most patients have studied their numbers and figured out what is coming next. Some thirty enzymes and chemicals are measured, each one interconnected to its cousins, each one a telltale sign for an organ or system inside the body. Each day, the numbers stretch across the yard-long chart, forming a continuum that allows trends and changes to be spotted easily. If certain numbers begin rising, that can be a sign of rejection. If kidney enzyme numbers rise, that can be a sign of too much immunosuppression damaging the kidneys. The trick for the surgeons is to find a balance—enough immunosuppression to ward off rejection without too much to kill the kidneys and invite infection. The trick is to find the natural balance; the problem is, of course, that the transplant is an unnatural act. Oblivious to the old margarine commercial (It's not nice to fool Mother

Nature . . .), the wall charts become a broad tableau on which this game of one-upping nature is played out.

Some patients, so fixated on the numbers that their lives revolve around the daily or weekly lab tests, have learned ways to tap into the hospital computer system and retrieve their numbers before they are posted. Sometimes they misread the numbers; more often they are prepared for good or bad news before the team ever arrives in the room for its look.

"How are your numbers today?" patients often ask each other. "Going down."

"That's good."

To Randy Roady, one number became the focus of his attention. His liver numbers were declining, meaning that the surgery to fix his bile duct was becoming less and less likely. But his red blood cell count was declining as well—not a good sign. He was losing blood, and he wasn't replacing it. For now, the team kept giving him bags of blood from the blood bank. So low was his blood that before a biopsy, they had to give him an extra blood transfusion in case he bled from the needle stuck into his liver. Biopsies can be messy affairs: A long, hollow needle is stuck into the side of the patient with only local anesthesia, and a sample of liver tissue is pierced and pulled out. The doctor with the needle is operating blindly, obviously, and occasionally one or two have missed the liver altogether. If they happen to hit a nerve on the way in, the pain can be intense. Patients understandably dread biopsies, which usually are infrequent but can come twice a week for a patient in trouble.

Each afternoon, rounds take the same course. The fellows and surgeon begin in X ray, checking the films. Then they go to the ICU, picking up other doctors, a nutritionist, a pharmacist, a coordinator, a research nurse, and sometimes even a chaplain and social worker. Then the team visits with families in the ICU waiting room, bolts down a corridor and up a flight

■

of stairs to the pathology lab to look at the day's biopsies under microscopes, and then heads to the fourteenth floor.

At pathology, they sit around a group microscope run by Weldon Tillery, the jovial and highly respected head of pathology at Baylor, and study swirls and paisleys of cells from liver tissue. Like Rorschach tests, the biopsy slides in the eyes of the untrained can look like anything the imagination can conjure. Tillery is the master of reading the slides. Whenever the team is befuddled, he can identify the strange patterns and come up with a guess, if not a diagnosis, of what the sample shows.

Randy Roady's liver was the first of ten biopsies one day—a marathon session in the formaldehyde-smelling pathology lab. "Overall, his biopsy looks very good. Occasional [rejection] cells start creeping in," Tillery muttered. "It's not that impressive, but it is more than you like to see. Then you get down here, and you get one that's more impressive. Here's one tract with ductal damage. I think it's portal reaction, probably early acute rejection."

"It's about the right time for it," Dale Distant noted. Eight days to two weeks out—prime rejection time.

On the screen, blue dots swarmed like an ant colony, surrounding cells for the kill. When foreign matter enters the human body, whether the virus of a common cold, or the bacteria of a scraped knee, or the liver of a transplant, the human immune system goes about attacking the invader and killing it. Lymphocytes—actually a subgroup of killer lymphocytes called T-cells—seek out the intruder cells and begin chomping on them, much like the Pac-Man video game. The process can be seen under a microscope when the patterns of attack are identified. If rejection is not reversed, it will destroy the liver and kill the patient. Statistically, sixty percent of the transplant patients have a bout with rejection. Those that do also end up having higher incidences of fungal and bacterial infections because their immune systems have to be suppressed even more.

■

The first line of defense against rejection is a course of megadoses of steroids—one huge burst tapered down over a week. If that doesn't work, a drug called OKT-3 is used, a magic bullet so powerful it knocks the patient into bed, sometimes even into cardiac arrest, but it usually kills the lymphocytes as well. OKT-3 is a monoclonal antibody—a high-tech, genetically engineered version of the body's own disease-fighting arsenal. It attacks and destroys the killer T-cell lymphocytes themselves. But it can be used only once in a patient's lifetime.

After OKT-3, if the patient is still rejecting, other drugs might be tried. But if those don't work, then the patient would probably need a new liver all over again. And the statistics get worse the more you talk about retransplanting. A few patients might need four livers before one works right.

Rejection—even the word sounds incredibly harsh to patients—is the thing all transplant patients fear most. Bo Husberg makes a conscious effort to call rejection "reaction," as in, "The biopsy confirms you are having a reaction." Doesn't sound as bad. Maybe to ease patient fears, they should call it something even more benign like "Medawar's Disease"—in honor of Sir Peter who first identified and described the immune system in the 1940s.

As complicated as reading the pathology slides can be, a simple rule is that blue cells (made blue by stains used to differentiate between types of cells) surrounded by blue cells is a bad sign. Red is good, blue within blue is bad.

Randy Roady had some bright blue within blue when his biopsy specimen slide was flashed on the screen.

Upstairs, Marlon Levy found himself sitting at the bedside again. Roady's numbers on the wall chart had actually come down that day, contradicting Tillery's diagnosis that the liver was rejecting. "The biopsy shows signs of rejection. It's not convincing enough to treat while your numbers are coming down."

■

"I feel ready to go shoot some pool," said Randy, his happy-go-lucky self slowly returning.

"I think you're better," Levy speculated.

"I feel better."

As he left the room, Marlon Levy shook his head and muttered to the team, "I'm surprised. Which one of you gave blood this morning for him?"

Almost as fast as Mel Berg was ushered into surgery November 5—two days after the national election—he was pulled out of the intensive care unit. The white-haired Floridian had lucked out as backup to the cancer patient. Now he was cruising through recovery. Concerns were small: a little too much fluid on his chest X ray, but not much else. Within thirty-six hours, he was out of the ICU and on his way to the fourteenth floor.

But there were reminders of just how sick transplant patients are made in order for a renewed life. On Sunday, Day Three post-transplant, the sixty-eight-year-old Berg threw up four times. He thought the world was coming to an end, and for the first time in years, he cried. The illness was terrifying to his family, but not even worrisome to Marlon Levy, who was doing rounds even though he had gone that night to retrieve the liver in El Paso for Don Bryan, and gone "vertical" just a few hours before Sunday rounds.

"He's not sleeping much, and he's got a lot of back pain. But he's a tough old coot," Rob Berg said.

Mel's kidney numbers were racing higher, indicating they were not at all pleased with the influx of FK 506. Especially in older people, the immunosuppressive drugs can be extremely toxic to the kidneys, raising the possibility of kidney failure right after surgery. Over the years, evidence has grown that cyclosporine and FK also raise the probability that liver-transplant patients will be back in five to ten years for a kidney transplant. Baylor was already seeing several of its first successful transplant patients under evaluation for new kidneys.

In Berg's case, the FK was reduced from twelve milligrams a day to eight to give his kidneys a break. It seemed to help, and recovery raced ahead. By Tuesday, sixty-eight-year-old Mel Berg was walking around the fourteenth floor, boasting about his five-day-old liver.

"This place is a miracle factory," Rob Berg marveled.

A routine biopsy yielded a textbook example of the perfect transplanted liver. "It looks as good as Madonna," someone remarked in the pathology lab. "Well, I don't know about that, guys, but it looks pretty darn good to me," Dr. Tillery said.

The next week, Bo Husberg was startled as he led the transplant team into a patient's room on rounds.

"There he is!" Don Bryan shrieked from his hospital bed. "There's a wonderful man. You made me feel like a million bucks."

"Well, I'll take half the credit. I'd like to feel like half a million," Husberg said.

"You're wonderful people. You really are," Bryan added.

After just two days in the intensive care unit, Don Bryan was up on the fourteenth floor. As sick as a person is made in an organ transplant, Bryan was already much better off than he was before. He was happy for the first time, relaxed for the first time, and terribly relieved to finally get a liver before it was too late.

"I can feel the difference. I don't know if that's just mental, but I really feel so much healthier," he said.

Healthy he hadn't been in a long time. The source of Bryan's liver cirrhosis was unknown, but he had been exposed to Benzene and Toluene, two toxic chemicals, when he worked in an American Petrofina refinery in Big Spring, Texas, not far from his farm. Don believed that had something to do with his illness.

On the farm, Bryan had had his share of setbacks, too. He and Cathy, his second wife who at forty-five is eighteen years younger, tried to start a vineyard only to learn at harvest time that the Lubbock, Texas, winery they contracted with had failed. They had lost two years of cotton crops to floods and had decided to quit the cotton business. Now they were working on an apple orchard. While Don was hospitalized, Cathy tried to keep the farm up long-distance from Dallas.

Bryan was recovering well. His small liver, the one from the tiny Hispanic woman, was struggling a bit with inflammation. Sonograms showed that flow through the liver was tough—there was a lot of resistance. But still, it was working well.

For Cathy, being at the hospital was a welcome change, even though some of the doctors seemed to stare at her, trying to figure out if she was wife or daughter since she looked so much younger than pallid Don. At her sister's house she had been nursing Don around the clock, cleaning urinals, forcing feedings, sitting up all night with the sleepless, sickly grump. "I was worn out, too," she said. "This is a big relief for me."

The first day after the transplant, Arden Lynn, who was still waiting after losing a liver that went to the woman in a coma, came down to Baylor to visit. Arden and the Bryans had become friends in evaluation, and now they were their own private support group. The strain of waiting clearly showed on Arden, saddening Cathy.

"She got all dressed up to come down here. It was a real struggle for her, and she put on a good face. But we've got to get a liver for Arden. People don't realize how sick she really is because she puts on such a good face."

Slowly, the shine began to fade from Don Bryan. All bones with no padding, he had a horrendous time during a

■

sonogram test, laid out on a cold stainless steel table. He was having spasms in his chest. His numbers had risen a bit, so a biopsy was scheduled. He was on the edge, normally nervous, now becoming more and more anxious, more and more agitated. Enrolled in a study of emotions the Baylor nurses were conducting, Don Bryan was already at the top of the anxiety charts, and he hadn't finished his first week yet.

Nights were far worse than days. One night, Don's ascites—the fluid in his abdomen that his liver had not yet been able to process—burst out through stitches when he rolled over in his sleep. The fluid wet the bed, spilled to the floor and drove Don into a panic.

Visits from other patients just added to his anxiety. Mel Berg came by often. "Look at how well he's doing—and he's older than me," Don would grumble. Berg was sixty-eight; Bryan sixty-three. Then there was Kelly Moore, the thirty-seven-year-old fellow West Texan who received the questionable fatty liver. He was up and around and doing great. They both got their livers before Don, and he remained bedridden and miserable. Don began to think more and more that things were not going well at all.

The numbers posted on the wall told a different story, however. "Who can argue with success?" Klintmalm asked as he stared at Bryan's wall chart. "Just plan on discharge next Monday if all goes as we hope. But you have to build up muscle mass."

Discharge? Don could barely make it to the bathroom.

Mel Berg's liver numbers started creeping up, although not as fast as his anxiety over them. Another biopsy again found no rejection, but the numbers kept going up. "We need to watch him closely. Something may be going on," Bo Husberg warned.

Within a week, Mel was shaky, worried, and anxious.

■

He had had a terrible night, up sick. Most of all, he was frightened.

"I know other people up here've got it worse than me, are worse off than me. But this has been rough, been hard, you know?" he said.

His anxiety wasn't matched by Klintmalm, however. "Everything looks perfectly fine," Klintmalm assured Berg. "Maybe home this week."

"Oh, thank you, doctor," Berg stammered.

Klintmalm had other worries than Mel Berg's anxiety. Another patient, Jo Ann Carroll, the woman who was found to have cancer in her bile duct as well as her liver, had suddenly taken a turn for the worse.

A favorite among the team, she had done well after the transplant. She had been personnel manager of a large Dallas-based chain of jewelry stores, with a warm, friendly husband and a couple of attentive daughters. Suddenly, however, she had begun to crash, almost inexplicably. As in Nora Barnes's case, the specialists all scratched their heads and pointed fingers the other way. As with Nora Barnes, she started with some twitching and seizures. It looked like neurological trouble, except nothing was found wrong; then lung trouble, except that nothing was found wrong; then heart trouble, except that nothing was found wrong.

"I'm afraid Carroll is going to die on us tonight," Klintmalm said to the team after rounds. "I get very bad vibes. Look how much worse she is in eight hours. Something is very wrong, and we don't know what it is. I'm very worried about her."

By Thursday, Don felt even worse. A note was stuck to the wall chart so it would not be missed by the team: "Pt. [patient] is miserable." The fluid had built around his belly, giving him that pregnant look again.

■

"I wanted so much to wake up with a flat belly," Don said. Mel Berg, in the room next door, was close to being discharged. He had his share of irritants and anxieties, but was up and about and walking the hospital corridors with gusto. Klintmalm was stressing exercise to Don, but he could barely walk. He tried climbing stairs, but couldn't make it, adding to his feeling of inadequacy. His abdomen leaked fluid again that night and leaked again during physical therapy, leaving a trail of ascites along the floor. The next night, he woke up with "the strangest sensation, prickly tingles. I thought I was dead, I really did. And I jumped out of bed," Don said. The patient was indeed miserable, and the only prescription the surgeons were offering, other than filling some liter-sized bottles with his belly fluid, was time.

"Everything is perfect," Klintmalm said after another glance at the latest numbers.

"I wish I could live up to that, but I don't feel as good as I look," Don said.

Actually, he looked terrible. Only his numbers looked good. He moaned when his tender abdomen was touched. He had a hacking cough that kept him, and Cathy, awake all night. He had a viral infection in his mouth. "I'm as miserable as I've ever been in my life," he groaned.

After more than a week in intensive care and two weeks on the fourteenth floor, Randy Roady was convinced he knew how the hospital worked. Whatever you did, they'd tell you that you were wrong. He took a shower one day and was scolded by a nurse for taking a shower. The next day, he found himself being scolded for not getting clean. He got out of bed one day, only to be ordered back. The next shift he was chastised for not getting out of bed.

"If you eat, they say, 'What are you eating? Who told

■

you to eat that?' And if you don't eat, they're all over you for not eating."

For the past two days, Randy, anxious to get out of the hospital, dressed each afternoon for rounds and made sure he was out of bed, in a chair, his suitcase packed and in his hand so the team would see him ready to go. Each time, the answer was not yet.

Now Randy Roady was hatching a plan to spring himself from the $1,000-per-day prison. It was Friday, and his kids were coming down from Oklahoma where they were staying with relatives so they could stay in school. A big weekend was planned, a triumphant weekend. After all the heartache, all the depression, all the pain and hurt, Randy not only was getting his life back, he was getting his kids back this weekend, too. So when the team came by Friday afternoon, Randy the schemer was shirtless and in bed, looking for all the world like a sickly hospital patient.

"Randy, what are you doing in bed?" Marlon Levy asked as he walked into the room.

"See," Randy said to Cynthy, confident that his trick was working. She couldn't keep from laughing.

"Get out of bed, Randy. Go to the apartment. Can you come in Sunday morning for lab work? We need to keep an eye on your kidneys."

"I'll deliver it personally. Let's have breakfast," an ebullient Randy said.

"Get out of here," Levy snickered.

The Roadys finished packing, taking down the cards, collecting the toothbrushes. In their excited haste, they forgot to take down the "Hurry Home" orange sign from Davis. Cynthy went off to get the pickup and park it out front. A nurse helped Randy onto the elevator and took him down to the first floor.

Suddenly, Randy felt light-headed. The elevator reached

■

the lobby, and the nurse had to tell Randy to get off. He got to the glass front door, saw his pickup, stopped and said to the nurse, "I'm not going to make it. We better go back up."

Then he fainted.

"I thought, This is it, it's all over. I'm not even going to live to get out this hospital door," Roady said later.

Back on fourteen, Randy began confessing. It turned out he had had excruciating pain in his abdomen all day, but had been afraid to tell anyone for fear of jinxing his weekend reunion. He thought it was just related to his constipation. "I didn't tell the doctors because I wanted to get out so bad," he said.

Dale Distant found that his vital signs were normal, and told him that he was probably just very dry because of all the powerful diuretics he had been given to rid his body of that sixty pounds of excess fluid. The pain seemed to be along the incision line, and that was OK, too. Now, after drying him out the past two weeks, they would have to pump him up with some fluids.

"What did he say?" a nurse came in to ask after Distant had left.

"He ordered me a case of Bud Light because I'm dry," Randy offered. "Dr. Levy's probably out there laughing hysterically at me now."

He wasn't.

Cynthy unpacked, and then decided to take down the "Hurry Home" banner, which suddenly seemed like a cruel reminder. The weekend with the kids would be in the hospital room. It was ironic, but it was the hospital room that was beginning to feel more like home than anything else.

It turned out that Randy Roady's hematocrit, the count of red cells in his blood, had dropped to a very low twenty-one percent at the time of his fainting. It had been twenty-nine percent, still low, and now was back to twenty-five percent after three more units of blood had been infused. Before he was going to get to try to leave again, transplant fellow Tom Renard suggested that the team spot him a "crit" of thirty percent.

An ultrasound exam, similar to the ultrasound used on pregnant women, had found no bleeding or pooling of blood in his belly the following Monday. Nothing could be found wrong, actually, except that his crit was low. He had been given a tremendous amount of blood in the operating room, Dale Distant noted, and his body was just working through that. The pain had lessened. If the hematocrit came up to thirty, Randy could go to the apartment in the morning.

"The question really is how far are we going to chase this? Should we do a CT scan? No," Bo Husberg told the team, then turned to Randy. "You would just be one phone call away, and you would not be alone. I think you can take it easy and give it a try."

Randy had changed. Now, instead of scheming to escape, he was scared to be discharged from the hospital. Suddenly, the fourteenth floor looked very safe. It is the nest, the place where people take care of you twenty-four hours a day. Now he was being told to fly on his own, and he wasn't sure if his wings would hold him.

"If they told me to stay, I really wouldn't mind. I want to make sure I'm strong enough to do this. Only thing is, when I do go out, I don't want to have to come back. That would crush me. I want to make sure I don't end up back here like the last time," he said.

On Tuesday, they told Randy at noon that he could go to the apartment, take it easy, call and come back if there was trouble. More tentative than the first time, he set out, made it into the apartment and tried to settle in. But by 10 P.M., he was running a high fever of 102.6. He called Transplant Services and was told to come back in—the answer he dreaded. His urine had turned tea colored. The pain in his abdomen was increasing. As before, he ended up back on fourteenth floor, more frustrated than ever.

Once again, Randy Roady was thinking about death. Death was something he lived with often. As a mortician, of course, and as a fireman, he responded to car crashes and house fires and once had to pull his cousin and nephew from a car wreck. Dead. Now it was weighing heavily on him. You think he might be used to it, hardened to it, but you never really get used to death. You block it out, you find ways to shield yourself, protect your sanity. But when it's you, what is there to shield yourself with? Randy Roady suddenly felt very naked, exposed, vulnerable. He was afraid he was dying. Twice he had been discharged and twice he had come back. At least the second time he made it beyond the front door. But more and more, it seemed as if he had two strikes against him.

The list of possible complications was expanding rapidly for Randy. He could be bleeding internally, he could be rejecting, he could have an infection. His numbers were going up—a bad sign. He had some fluid in his belly, dots scattered around like a chain of islands on a map. And his chest X ray showed something else—he also might have pneumonia. A long, hushed discussion took place on rounds under Roady's wall chart, while Randy and Cynthy tried to eavesdrop as best they could. "What is that?" she asked a couple of times, trying unsuccessfully to get in on the discussion. The case was recounted: the story of the donor with vegetation on the heart valve, thus putting Roady on an antibiotic, Cipro, as a preventative. He had rejection earlier, but was not treated because his numbers had gone down. There had been concern about his bile duct, but they didn't do anything because his numbers had gone down. Where was the answer?

Quickly, Cynthy was coming to the realization that the surgeons are really just men and women trying to stretch the bounds of medicine, just people working hard who don't have all the answers. After all the dazzle and glory, it turns out they're just people struggling to do the right thing, people who make mistakes, guess wrong, run into trouble. Sometimes they win, sometimes, it turns out, they lose. All of a sudden came the realization that they don't have all the answers. My God, they don't know what's wrong with my husband. They don't know how to fix it. They can fix anything, I thought. She sat in a chair, curled up in a shell-like protective mode. Randy was depressed, a victim of high expectations and too many disappointments. Her children were worried and disappointed that daddy was still in the hospital. Now, there was aggravation, too.

"They don't talk to you," she said, annoyed, frustrated, and more than anything, scared.

A pool of blood was found in Randy's belly and sucked out with a needle. It was sent off to be cultured for infections. Husberg poked his chest and declared the pain lessened because "You don't hit me when I do this."

His liver biopsy looked pretty good—especially better than the biopsy seen the same day that had a strange, spongy-type area in it that Tillery teased the team about. "Oh my God, look at that," he declared, a smile on his lips with his eyes planted in the microscope. The doctors never saw the smile, their eyes fixed in their own microscopes. "Bo, how's this patient doing?"—adding to the team's sudden tension. "I haven't seen this in years. . . ."

"The patient is fine, I think," Husberg replied, without much confidence.

"Bo," Tillery said, his smile curling out from under his microscope, "There's a piece of cotton in this liver, because this is a cotton fiber off a sponge or something." Fortunately, there is no danger from cotton in the liver.

With Cynthy scowling at the team, arms crossed, the doctors launched into another discussion at the wall chart altar in Roady's room. His bile duct was OK, his biopsy was OK, so there was no rejection. His numbers had come down—but just a bit. There was no bacteria growing in the blood that had been drawn out of his chest. So what was wrong? A virus could explain the numbers and the fever. Maybe it was a virus that the body had taken care of itself?

"I like to hear that," Randy chimed in.

"So are you going home soon?" asked Michelle Long, the social worker.

"Don't say those words," Randy shot back.

A dozen days after the surgery, Mel Berg was scared. He was told he'd be going home soon to his apartment at Twice Blessed House, having breezed through the process better than most of those half his age. Still, Mel's family was worried it was too much too soon.

"If he doesn't feel better tomorrow, he's not going any-more," his wife Connie insisted. Clinically, though, everything was looking good for Berg.

"Out tomorrow," Klintmalm told him.

"Oh my God, that's fast. Thirteen days. Is that too fast?"

In support group, Mel became star of the show. "I never thought I'd make it here to this meeting," he said. "I'd given up hope that I'd ever get a liver." He was so sick before, in fact, that his sons thought when he left Florida, they'd never see him alive again. Now there he was, dapper and trim, dazzling the support group with a record-breaking recovery.

"I don't care about the holidays this year. There's plenty of time ahead next year for Thanksgiving and Christmas." It seemed like an odd, if not bold, statement from a sixty-eight-year-old liver transplant patient. But there was no holding back Mel Berg now.

Later that day, Mel Berg was discharged, thirteen days

■

after his transplant, a week before Thanksgiving. He shook hands with Klintmalm, and offered thanks. "I'm amazed, just amazed," he said.

He didn't know it, but the next day Eugene Konecci, the cancer patient who missed out on the liver Berg received, died in Austin. He was sixty-seven.

The longer nothing terribly wrong was found, the better Randy Roady's spirits became. As another weekend approached, a big weekend when the kids were coming down and Randy's preacher would be visiting, Roady returned to his schemes, sitting in a chair near the wall chart during rounds, covering his mouth and saying, in a deep, muffled, authoritarian, medical-type voice, "I think we can send him home. Yes, you're right. I think we can send him home."

Tomorrow, the answer came. Maybe Sunday.

Sunday brought release, but again Randy was far from happy.

"It's hard to leave this time," he said. "I don't have much confidence. It's tough to leave the nest after so many disappointments."

On Tuesday, he was checked in the weekly clinic as scheduled, and felt horrible.

"I feel worse than before the surgery," he said in the hospital cafeteria after clinic, so weak he was barely able to lift the Styrofoam cup of ice in front of him. "I'm sick to my stomach. I can't eat. I can't sleep. I'm irritable. I snapped at Cynthy twice. I'm uncomfortable with these staples in me. I felt much better the first week after I got out of the ICU. This is really strange.

"If I feel this bad tomorrow, I won't go to support group."

That day at lunch, fellows Lars Backman, Tom Renard,

and Dale Distant got together for a freebie meal from a drug company. As they often do, they end up chatting about patients, comparing notes, razzing each other over the condition of their patients. If the patient doesn't do well, then the fellow who transplanted the liver is in for some ribbing.

"Did Randy Roady make it to clinic today?" one asked.

"Just barely," Distant said, ready for the ridicule. "He's not looking good. The anastomosis is OK, it's the envelope [the body] that's shit."

The next day, Randy was back in the hospital, unable to eat and feeling terrible. The liver was OK, apparently, but the package around it, the envelope, was indeed shit. He was dry again, so there would be more fluid and more blood. And maybe he had a bleeding ulcer? They would check for that.

A nurse came into Randy's room with scorn. "You? Back! I told you not to come back," she jabbed. "If you go home this weekend, I *don't* want to come in Monday and find you in one of these rooms!"

The fourteenth floor was full by the time it was Klintmalm's turn to lead rounds again, and it seemed ironic because the team had gone almost two weeks without a transplant. Some longtime patients had come in, some had never left, and several rooms were taken by extremely ill people on the waiting list, so sick they had to be hospitalized. Despite the priority they commanded on the list, there were no livers. "It's been a disaster," Klintmalm announced at his weekly staff meeting. "Anybody know where we can find a donor?"

Randy Roady, who never made it out of the hospital for the weekend, was curled in bed covered with blankets. It had been four weeks since his transplant, and Thanksgiving was fast approaching. A bleeding ulcer was ruled out, and now the theory that a virus was at work was being explored.

■

Next door, a kidney transplant recipient was also curled up looking sick.

"Well, my dear. You look like you feel like *sheet* today," Klintmalm said.

Down the hall, the whacked-out liver recipient who had begun confessing to child abuse while drugged was now on the floor, still disoriented but better medically.

"There's just one thing I'm concerned about," he barked to the team, catching their attention quickly. "I'm really concerned about this, and no one else seems to be concerned about it . . .

"There's this contest, this lottery, the new Texas lottery. What if I've won, and nobody checks for me? That's the money I'm going to pay you with."

Everyone pushed and shoved to get out of the room before they burst out laughing. As the herd thundered to the hallway, the man's mother was heard assuring her confused son.

"Oh honey, don't worry. Dr. Klintmalm isn't concerned about the money."

More laughter.

With Thanksgiving two days away, the question became once again, why keep Randy in the hospital?

"I see nothing wrong, but I hate to keep sending you home only to have you come back," Klintmalm said. "But it's crazy to keep you here waiting for something to happen."

Then, turning to Cynthy, he tried a new theory: "Could it be your cooking?"

"Don't give him any ideas," she shot back.

"We'll plan to send you home tomorrow."

With family and friends all headed down from Davis for Thanksgiving at the Roady's Twice Blessed House apartment, Randy was discharged Wednesday. Thanksgiving would certainly be special this year. Despite all the woes, there was a lot to be thankful for.

■

• • •

For Thanksgiving, the Bergs joined a community celebration at Twice Blessed House organized by volunteers from the Junior League. Each family brought their turkey-day specialty. For Connie, it was candied yams. For Mel, it was all a miracle.

"I'm doing so good it's scary," Berg said. "It seems like a dream. I look at Don Bryan and I'm so thankful I'm doing well."

At the apartment, Connie fell ill and Mel, the patient, ended up nursing her all night, reminding her every now and then that it was supposed to be the other way. He began to plan a return to his golf club business. He started tinkering around Twice Blessed House, fixing a broken lamp, fixing a broken door bell, searching for other projects.

Thanksgiving simply brought more worry for Don Bryan, still in the hospital. Any celebration was out of the question, and now Don's numbers were going up. A biopsy showed questionable rejection—"?rej." it said on the wall chart, employing the question-mark diagnostic tool. There was inflammation in the liver and possible early-stage rejection. But Don was too weak to tolerate even the mildest treatment for rejection—the "recycle" of megadoses of steroids. To avoid that trauma, Bob Goldstein, back from his mountain-climbing adventure in Nepal, decided on a shot here and a shot there of solumedrol— a potent steroid that can hinder the rejection process in the liver.

The numbers kept going up. "If they're up again tomorrow," Goldstein warned, "we'll have to give you a full steroid recycle, and I really don't want to do that. It's a lot of steroids. But if we have to, we have to."

"Am I in trouble?" Don asked, his voice shaking.

• • •

■

For a change, Randy Roady felt good enough to stay out of the hospital for more than twenty-four hours. Cynthy drove to Davis to pick up their children, and Randy's brother and his family came down for Thanksgiving. It was one of those wonderful family days, simple, joyful, crowded, and hectic.

But it was also short-lived. By Friday night, Randy was throwing up and back up on the fourteenth floor, where he remained all weekend. "This one was very upsetting to the kids because they saw it all," he said.

Actually, five patients had come in Friday night from Twice Blessed House, all throwing up. Too much turkey? Food poisoning? Perhaps. More likely, a virus was going around.

So by Monday morning, Randy was given the all-clear once again. Go home, for the fifth time.

He got as far as the front desk nurses station. "You can't leave," Lars Backman bellowed in his Pavarotti voice. "Your blood count is too low."

Randy simply turned around and headed back down the hall.

Finally, the team was beginning to ask the question Cynthy had been pondering all along. Where was the blood going? They think he's not bleeding. He didn't throw up any blood. There's no blood in his urine or stool. What's happening to it? "Maybe it's because they keep drawing so much for all these tests," Randy speculated.

Not even out of the hospital yet, the bills were stacking up at the apartment. Baylor sent an $81,000 bill for the time in the intensive care unit and the operating room. Doctors sent bills. Transplant Services billed for its flat $20,000 fee. There were bills for lab tests, X rays, and the organ bank procurement charges. Already, Randy had hit $160,000. Already, Oklahoma Blue Cross/Blue Shield had declared it would not pay all of Klintmalm's Transplant Services bill, setting up a fight over that.

"It's unbelievable. If the insurance doesn't pay it, I'd just say, 'You can have me. Take your liver back.' "

The tension was wearing on everyone. Cynthy had dropped the kids off at school before heading for Dallas and ended up in a huge, tearful scene. It seemed as though the kids were getting more and more distant.

And by now, the transplant team had gone from gods to garage mechanics. "They're just trying different things until they find the problem and can fix it," Randy said. "Maybe they're right. Maybe I have a really big problem. Maybe it is my wife's cooking."

"I thought we sent Randy home?" Glen Hansen, a surgical resident, asked as the team entered the room.

"Randy had a crit of nineteen," Bob Goldstein responded.

"So what's his crit now?"

"Twenty."

"Where's it going?" Hansen asked.

"That's what we want to know," Cynthy fumed.

Dale Distant wanted to start Roady on an antiviral medication because cultures might not turn positive for a full month. The battery of testing started all over again. Check for a bleeding ulcer. Biopsy the liver. Ultrasound and CT scan.

"We're worried there still may be some bleeding internally," Goldstein said. "We're worried this could be a virus."

They reduced his FK—his primary immunosuppression medication—to give his body's own immune system a better chance of fighting off whatever was attacking him. The tradeoff is that reducing the FK can raise the risk of rejection.

"I confess. I'm selling the blood," Randy yelled as the team left.

"Randy. Randy. Randy," Hansen laughed, shaking his head.

The team had lost another patient, Jo Ann Carroll, the

■

190

woman who was found to have cancer in her bile duct, as well as her liver. She had begun to crash inexplicably the same way as Nora Barnes, twitching and seizures while specialists all scratched their heads. Then she lingered for several weeks in the ICU. Still puzzling all who studied her, Jo Ann Carroll died. "Her two biggest diagnostic risks," Dale Distant lamented, "were that she was a very nice lady with a very nice family." It was a popular refrain: The nice ones never get a break.

Like Nora Barnes, an autopsy on Jo Ann Carroll found nothing wrong. The mystery heightened anxiety. Compassion levels were low through the week.

After more than five weeks in and out of the hospital, Randy Roady was actually improving again, and the doctors finally got a break. One test came back positive, indicating the probability of a drug reaction. That might explain it all: Something Randy was taking was making him sick and was attacking his blood.

"Stop the Flexril. Stop the Bactrim. Stop the Vancomyacin," barked Goldstein. Finally, someone was able to take some action after weeks of simple head scratching.

"Why is he on Cipro?" The story of the vegetation on the heart valve incident while he had been on Mount Everest was recalled. It was a mandatory two-month course, the team told him. GK said so.

"Stop it. How's that?" Goldstein said with a smile. "The cultures were all negative. He's been on it long enough."

At their feet in front of the wall chart was a fully packed suitcase, sitting there on the floor.

"Is this a hint?" Goldstein asked. "He's been back and forth so much, I hate to keep him going back and forth."

A pharmacist reminded Goldstein that it could take a week for the effects of the medications to wear off and give a clear indication whether that was indeed the problem.

"Keep him," he said, then turned to Randy and Cynthy.

"We may have to give you blood tonight. I hate to send you home and have you come right back."

"We're used to it," Cynthy said.

As the team left, Randy fumed. "Get that bitch's name who talked him out of it," he said.

One day later, the theory was already changing. "It's acting viral," Goldstein said. "Have we checked his hepatitis B and C? We need to do that. He's two months out, and we need to start probing more."

At last, Don Bryan could go up some stairs, and walk around the hospital floor. He was developing a bit of strength and getting a bit of encouragement. His numbers had bounced around, up and down, enough to keep Bob Goldstein from calling for a full steroid recycle, and the strategy appeared to be paying dividends. Don was getting stronger, sleeping, eating.

"For every two good days, I get hit with a bad one," he said. "I start thinking, here it comes."

He usually was right about that. One morning he woke up in a pool of uncontrollable sweat at 7 A.M. "I felt worse than I *ever* felt," he said. "I thought I was dead. I just thought, this is it. I give up. I can't stand any more. I give up."

"We're not ready to give up yet," Cathy insisted. "We're going to hang in there a little longer."

The episode was most likely a reaction to the steroids he was taking, and further evidence that a big dose of steroids would really knock Don back. Still, the question-mark rejection had not been resolved. On rounds, his numbers were down a bit, but so was the level of cyclosporine in his blood—another sign of rejection, an indication that his body was not absorbing much of the antirejection medication. Goldstein ordered more cyclosporine, and someone asked about a steroid recycle.

"I really don't want to put him on a steroid recycle," Goldstein insisted.

■

Don, flat on his back, flashed a two-finger V-for-victory salute to Goldstein, who smiled, saluted Don, and walked out.

The next day, team was greeted by another note on the wall in Don Bryan's room.

"1) Regular diet instead of soft food?

"2) Staples out?"

"Sick of the baby food?" Goldstein asked.

"You goddamn right about that!" Bryan said with gusto.

"Sounds like he's doing better," Tom Renard chuckled softly to the wall chart.

Don had walked four times that day. The fluid in his belly had diminished. Talk of having to send him to a rehabilitation facility was diminishing. His numbers were going down. Even though his surgical buddies, including Kelly Moore, had all been discharged, his spirits were improving. Things were looking up, finally.

"Looks like we're going in the right direction," Goldstein said.

"I'm climbing that mountain with you, Doc," said Don, well aware of Goldstein's exploits.

Don was doing so well that he had begun to complain about the hospital food. "Would you eat this?" he asked a nurse one day. She said "no," and gave him a menu for a Chinese take out/delivery service.

Each night during the week, Randy Roady had been spiking temperatures over 100, some to 102. The possibility of recurrent hepatitis became more plausible. Was it possible he got something new from all the blood transfusions, or from the liver itself?

"I've got to get out of this hospital. I've just got to get

■

out," Randy sighed, acting more and more like a caged animal. "I'm bored. I'm going crazy here. I better be out by Christmas so I can at least go home for the day."

Blood was found in his urine, for no apparent reason. Rather than good news, this seemed to just deepen the mystery.

"We have to wait for the medication levels to go down and correct the red blood cell problem. If that doesn't correct it, then it's something else," Goldstein told him.

For the first time, Randy sneered as they left. "I feel fine except I'm a prisoner here and I'm paying for it. I can't get out. Why do I have to stay, just to give blood every day?"

The floor was emptying out, with eight people discharged Friday afternoon, the weekend before Klintmalm's famous Swedish Christmas glögg party. Randy had renamed himself "NoGo" Roady, and NoGo now had almost an entire wing of the floor to himself.

"What's going on with NoGo Roady?" Goldstein asked.

Randy, his hematocrit only up to twenty-two, but rising on its own for a change, moved to the middle of the group, acting like one of the doctors on rounds.

"Look at that. Hmmmm," he said, fingers on chin and a puzzled look on his face.

"If we let you go, would you come in tomorrow and get a hematocrit count?"

"OK! Yes sir."

"And take your temperature tonight? It was 101 last night. You were supposed to go twenty-four hours without a temperature, you goofball. . . . Go home."

Randy beamed as he packed. "This will be my first weekend out. First weekend in almost two months. The kids are coming tonight . . .

"We're going to go buy a Christmas tree and put it up. We're going to have the best time."

NoGo, renamed "IGo," made nine patients discharged in one day. That tied the record.

■

• • •

Just when it looked as if Don Bryan had turned the corner, his roller coaster ride headed south again. His numbers shot up on Friday, the day of Randy Roady's discharge.

"Well, that's it. Turn me over and put me in the grave. I'm rejecting," he said after the team had delivered the bad news. A biopsy was ordered right away, and a steroid recycle was readied. Now, Goldstein had suggested, Don was much better prepared for it than the previous week. Stringing him along with injections of solucortef and solumedrol had bought some valuable time.

The biopsy Friday night was labeled "reg.??"—it didn't look any worse than the previous biopsy. So the same decision was made: Don would get a recycle only if his numbers go up Monday.

At rounds Monday, Tillery pulled out the weekend biopsies and said he had gone back to review them. First up: Don Bryan.

"This is the guy who every biopsy looks like rejection and Bob was pussyfooting around," said Tom Gonwa, the kidney expert attached to the team.

Marlon Levy, leading rounds that week, peered into the microscope.

"Oh shit," he said as Tillery pointed out the signs of rejection.

"I can argue with you, with Goran, with Bo," Gonwa said to Levy. "But with Bob, I know when to pick a fight and when not to pick a fight."

On the television screen hooked up to the microscope so that the entire team can see the biopsies, clear patterns of blue cells within rings of blue cells were found, like a snake strangling a rat before eating it.

"You can take a picture of that and put it in a textbook," Levy agreed.

"You just can't treat acute cellular rejection with solucortef," Gonwa said.

■

195

As the team entered Don Bryan's room, Lars Backman had the preprinted order sheet in his hand for a steroid recycle.

"We reviewed the biopsy," Levy began telling Bryan. "And some areas look worrisome for rejection."

Bryan suddenly looked shell-shocked.

Then, Dale Distant interrupted Levy. "His liver numbers are down, his cyclosporine level is up, his kidneys are tolerating it. I'd keep him where he is."

Levy looked. "No changes," he said.

Backman, shaking his head incredulously, put the recycle order sheet back in his holster.

"We'll wait another day and see how the liver is doing," Levy said, making the same decision Goldstein had made all the previous week.

Randy Roady's first weekend out was indeed the best ever. The family, reunited, decorated a Christmas tree in the apartment and celebrated the future, finally. When it was time to drive the kids back home to Oklahoma, Randy rode as far as the state line, meeting relatives there for a handoff and playfully touching his toe across the line into Oklahoma. "It was just great," he bubbled.

Monday morning Randy went up to the fourteenth floor voluntarily to check on the condition of a patient he had befriended, Bobby Zanders. Zanders was a twenty-two-year-old kid from Jim Thorpe, Pennsylvania, who had picked up hepatitis while stationed in the Pacific with the army. During his discharge physical in San Diego, doctors discovered poor liver function—so poor he needed a transplant right away. The army shipped him off to San Antonio, where a new military liver transplant program was underway, and he got a new liver.

But the job wasn't done all that well, and complications soon developed. Zanders was rejecting so much that the magic-bullet medication, OKT-3, which is only supposed to be used

■

once in a lifetime, was tried twice. Infection spread through the lower half of his body so deeply that doctors scraped away tissue virtually down to the bone.

Then, tossing their hands to the air in frustration, the army shipped Zanders to Baylor, hoping he might be able to get FK 506, which might be his only chance at reversing the rejection. That was in February, ten months before.

But Bobby Zanders was caught in one of those incredible bureaucratic, Congressional snafus, the kind that lead to scandals, the kind that kill people. His insurance through the military was with CHAMPUS, the government insurance agency. CHAMPUS (Civilian Health And Medical Program of the Uniformed Services) had a rule, actually handed down by Congress: No "experimental" medications were ever to be used. If they were, the patient would lose all his health insurance for the rest of his life. It was a horrifying version of the old Jack Benny joke: "Your money or your life."

It wasn't even a question of money to CHAMPUS, either. FK 506, still considered experimental because it had not yet received Food and Drug Administration approval, was free to all who took it. Fujisawa Pharmaceutical Corporation, the Japanese drug company that manufactures it, can't charge until it's approved. Yet rather than allow Bobby Zanders to get FK, CHAMPUS was most likely facing the prospect of paying for another transplant, and many more months of hospitalization, for Zanders. It wasn't a question of money. There was a rule, a law, and no exceptions could be made. No exceptions could be made for Bobby Zanders.

"CHAMPUS is so far out, they are literally condemning patients to death for no valid reason," Klintmalm said. "It's criminal. It's criminal. There's absolutely no justification for it. We've been talking with them for years about this, and the medical director at CHAMPUS agrees with us. But Congress has to change the law."

At Baylor, Klintmalm did all he could for Zanders: He

■

got him another liver. This one worked better than the first transplant, but still had its problems. By December, Zanders's body was attacking his bile ducts, and the only solution once again was another liver, a third transplant. That had come Thanksgiving weekend. But the newest liver brought more of the same, rejection and infection. There were problems sewing together Zanders's bile duct, and he had to be taken back to the operating room for a fix. There were problems with the fix, and now, Zanders was too far gone for a fourth transplant. Word spread through Twice Blessed House that weekend that Bobby Zanders, everybody's friend, was in serious trouble. Forget the insurance, forget the laws, the family pleaded. Give him FK. But it was too late, and not possible anyway without someone going to prison. Over the next twenty-four hours, Bobby Zanders would either turn the corner, or die.

Why, his mother asked Chaplain Grady Hinton. Why would God let this happen? Why would they go through this hell if the end result was that he died. He should have died ten months earlier without all this suffering. Why?

In his younger days, Chaplain Hinton would have tried to come up with an explanation to console the family, some theological theory that would offer compassion and maybe even hope. But Hinton had seen too much. Bad things do happen to good people.

Why?

Because.

Sometimes the gods won't be fooled. That's the only answer: there is no answer. You never know until you fight, and you fight knowing you may lose.

"How is Bobby Zanders?" Randy Roady asked a nurse on the fourteenth floor that Monday morning.

"He died yesterday."

"I think maybe it's a blessing," Randy said, a touch of anger in his voice. "I couldn't go through three of these. I couldn't do it.

■

"I think there are better places than this, you know? There are better places to be than this, and he deserves to be there."

By early December, Don Bryan was up and about, walking, climbing, talking a bit. His numbers were so good that Levy began cutting back his cyclosporine. A question remained: If he had been rejecting, then he should be placed on "triple therapy"—cyclosporine, steroids, and Imuran.

Before cyclosporine was discovered, Imuran, the anti-inflammatory drug, was the best antirejection medicine there was.

"Are we going to say he rejected and should be on triple therapy?" Levy asked the team. "Since we didn't shit or get off the pot. That's what Dick Nixon said in his first post-Watergate interview, you know. 'Shit or get off the pot.' It's true."

Two visitors came by to see Don while the team was in his room, but Don was gone, off walking somewhere.

"I don't know where he is, but he looks good, on paper at least," Levy told the Bryan neighbors from Big Spring.

Stumping away like Pooh, wearing the Mickey Mouse tie given to him by two patients who tried in vain to get him a Goofy tie, Marlon Levy offered one more wisecrack: "Good on paper, but I guess he looks kind of thin in person."

It had been thirty days since Don Bryan checked in to Baylor, and he finally got to see a bit of the outside world: He sneaked into the parking garage for a minute. All week the team had been preparing him for discharge Friday, it was even penciled on his chart. But there was no excitement for Don, only anxiety, even depression. Once again, he was scared. Like all the others, leaving the nest was terrifying.

"It's been a long haul," was about all he would mutter.

Like most patients, he had become fixated on his daily

numbers. He grew so anxious about the numbers that his wife found him one day weighing himself on a scale, jumping up and down and screaming, "My numbers are all wrong! MY NUMBERS ARE ALL WRONG!"

When Friday came, and the word was officially delivered that he could go to Twice Blessed House, Don Bryan looked crushed. He weakly shook hands with nurse Janel McDonald and Lars Backman, hiked up the falling pants of his crimson jogging suit, and slowly toddled out with all the spunk of a condemned man.

Five days later, he was back. This time, Don was acting completely muddled, as if his brain was not all there. Sitting in front of a fire over the weekend at his sister-in-law's house, he had taken some family pictures and just tossed them into the fire. He had taped over mirrors in the apartment because he couldn't stand to look at his stick-figure body, which had sunk to 123 pounds and not recovered much. He was having bathroom accidents and had started reciting "magic numbers." At wit's end, Cathy brought him back in, terrified that Don had suffered brain damage.

After CT scans of his head and psychiatric consultations, the conclusion was simply that Don Bryan was depressed. After being so down before the surgery, only to find that the miracle was slower and more painful than he had prepared for, the entire ordeal was too much, too debilitating, too frustrating. Perhaps because of the steroids he was taking, Don's brain was not working as it should.

"Will this go away, and he'll get better?" Cathy Bryan asked Bo Husberg after he explained the damage the steroids can do.

"We think so, that there's better than a fifty-fifty chance. But I can't guarantee it," Husberg said. "Only God knows."

It was the first time God had ever been mentioned by the team. In need of a little picker-upper, Don was started on

■

200

antidepression medication, Haldol. The next day, he was working out at Baylor's Tom Landry Sports Medicine Center, climbing stairs in the hospital, and smiling again. Husberg discharged him, and, one week before Christmas, Don set off in search of the best chicken-fried steak in Dallas.

Randy Roady celebrated his thirty-ninth birthday a day early, on a Sunday. He didn't have a pass from the doctors, but he went home to Davis anyway to take the children back to school. Sunday night, he sneaked into church late. Somebody was sitting in his regular seat, so he stayed in the back.

"The preacher looked up and said, 'Oh my God! Randy Roady's here.'

"It was the best birthday present ever, even better than the VCR from my mother-in-law."

Randy got a new pair of jeans, size thirty-six, down from size forty. He and Cynthy busied themselves with Christmas decorations and hunted for the best Christmas lights in Dallas. His hematocrit was up a point. Dale Distant asked him in clinic if he was still having fevers, then caught himself: "You wouldn't tell me if you were."

Except for the threatening letters that were already arriving from doctors' bill collectors, sent before the doctors had even filed claims with his insurance company, life was looking a whole lot better to Randy Roady.

Ten days later, Randy was home for Christmas. He went by City Hall to pal around with his buddies, and word spread through town. The *Davis News* got a picture of the reunion and put it on the front page: "A Visitor More Special Than Santa," it said.

"At Thanksgiving, he was pretty sick and I had my doubts that he'd be home for Christmas. But it turned out to be the best Christmas ever," Cynthy said.

On television they watched Randy's favorite movie,

"It's a Wonderful Life." Randy got socks, Nikes, clothes, and a new watch. His fourteen-year-old daughter, Heather, gave him a medical kit. Heath, his son, got an entire Raiders outfit—jacket, pants, shirt, etc. The Los Angeles Raiders are the coolest team logo to wear in junior high, even if it was the year the Dallas Cowboys made it to the Super Bowl. Randy was so excited about the whole thing that he forgot whether he took his evening dose of FK, and ended up calling Baylor in a panic at 11:45 P.M. Christmas Eve, asking what he should do.

But it was all working out. It was all looking as if it was indeed going to be a wonderful life for Randy Roady.

"Allow me to introduce my husband," Cathy Bryan beamed to Lars Backman at the first day of clinic after Christmas. "I got my husband back for Christmas."

Actually, it was Christmas Eve. Since the beginning Cathy had worried that Don was not nearly as sharp mentally as he had been before he got sick. His answers to questions were usually "yes" or "no." He was confused, disoriented, not tracking very well. There was no attention span at all. Don, a voracious reader and quick wit, hadn't read a word. He couldn't even concentrate enough to watch television. He just was not all there.

Then, on Christmas Eve, Cathy was talking about going home for a weekend to visit the farm in January. Usually in discussions of time, everything to Don was September—that was the month they came to Baylor. It was as if in Don's head, someone had smashed and broken the clock on September, and now everything was dated September.

"Well, it's December, so that's not too far," Don declared.

Cathy was floored. Don was beginning to make sense of the world around him in ways he hadn't since before the transplant. He had been switched from Haldol to Ritalin, a stimulant that gives the brain a jolt to help it focus, and suddenly he could compare blood pressure and temperature readings with Mel Berg and chat about the holidays. He picked up pamphlets in the clinic waiting room and started reading about liver disease.

Then, after grumbling that he had spent all the damn time in that hospital that he cared to and it was time to go, Don Bryan set out on a victory tour to the fourteenth floor. He was an instant hit, and somehow, he wanted to linger for a couple of hours.

"I want to apologize for everything I may have said," he proclaimed, hugging nurses.

None realized he was so tall. It was the first time they had seen Don Bryan standing up straight. From 123 pounds, he had filled out to 147, still barely covering his six-feet-two-inch frame. He paraded around the transplant unit looking quite dapper in a cap, suspenders, khakis, and L.L. Bean lace-up moccasins. When a physical therapist walked by, Don tried to hide against the wall. "I used to hate to see you coming," he joked. Grady Hinton, the chaplain, stopped the Bryans in the hall, too.

"I got my Christmas wish, I got my husband back," Cathy said.

"I knew all along he'd come back," Hinton boasted.

"Sure wish you had told me," Don cracked.

Then, in an ironic twist probably possible only in a transplant ward, Don Bryan went to visit Kelly Moore.

Moore, the American Airlines employee from Midland who had befriended Don after their transplants the same weekend and who had frustrated Don by bouncing back so quickly while Don struggled, had blown out his hepatic artery completely. It exploded, leaving his liver with blood supply only from the vein. Why it happened was unknown. Maybe because it was such a bad, fatty liver to begin with? Maybe fate? Maybe just very, very bad luck. But now Kelly Moore was sick in a hospital bed, dying, relisted on the waiting list, a high priority for another liver.

"I can't believe it," Don said over and over. "It breaks your heart."

What a tricky business.

CHAPTER 11

THE NUMBERS GAME II

O f all the many great mysteries of transplantation, from secrets of the body and mind to riddles of science and technology, one question has continuously confounded researchers:

What does it really cost?

Not what do the hospitals, labs, and doctors charge. Patients quickly learn that, as complicated bills pile up even before some are out of the intensive care unit. And not what do the insurance companies and government programs really pay, almost never the same as what is actually charged, leaving a debt for the patient to settle. No, the unanswerable question is one few, if any, hospitals ever reveal: How much profit is there in it?

The best guess so far: A lot.

The question is not simply one of curiosity. For the patients, the numbers posted on the wall chart twice a day are a source of grave concern, but the numbers that pile up in the mailbox can be a source of even greater worry. Bills run in five and six digits. Twenty thousand dollars for the surgeon's fee. One hundred two thousand dollars for the first portion of the hospital stay. What if the insurance company doesn't pay? What if the insurance company pays only a bit? What if I exceed my lifetime limit and lose my insurance forever? Is my life really worth $500,000? What kind of burden might I leave

■

behind for my family? Add to that the worry of another $1,000 per month in expenses for the cocktail of drugs needed to keep liver transplant patients alive, and soon money becomes so grave a concern that patients begin placing their own price on their lives.

After raising $150,000 for a liver transplant, one uninsured patient at Baylor saw his bills top $300,000 because he was not doing well. Still far from recovery, he asked that his feeding tube be removed because he didn't want to bankrupt his family. After a moving heart-to-heart talk with social worker Michelle Long and an assurance from Alison Victoria, the transplant program's financial administrator, that the hospital would work with him on the debt and promised not to force him to sell his house, the patient fought on.

And for the hospitals, and society, the question is a serious one since people are routinely turned away because they can't pay the price. But what if the price were thirty percent lower? Would more people survive the "wallet biopsy" test and have a chance at a life-saving transplant? Hospitals usually provide some token of transplantation care to the uninsured and poor and argue, as well, that were the service not profitable, it would drain resources from other departments and limit the care provided to the community in other ways. But is it also possible that nonprofit hospitals, at a time when all hospitals must cut costs, are turning away and letting die patients for the sake of profits—or "surpluses," as they are called at nonprofit institutions like Baylor?

The questions strike at the heart of health care reform. When Medicare, the program that provides health care coverage to the elderly, pays $200,000 for a patient to have a liver transplant, or pays $200 million for 1,000 patients to have liver transplants, the money comes straight out of taxpayers' pockets. In 1990, the federal Health Care Financing Administration, which handles Medicare claims, paid out $10 million for adult liver transplants, the most expensive of all transplant procedures. Just three years later, by 1993, the spending for livers climbed to $85 million and was projected to grow to $120 million in 1994—all of which makes it a very big, big-ticket item. Have we come to a public policy point where painful choices must be made? Would that $120 million be better spent immunizing all children against disease? The mystery remains to figure out how much the health care really costs and whether the price tag could be cut without injuring care. It's hard to make good public policy with bad data or even no data.

Transplantation is just a small slice of the nation's medical bill and a prime example of why costs are skyrocketing, a microcosm of a bigger issue as promising but expensive care is extended through technological advances to a wider population, including the elderly. As a big-ticket, high-risk procedure, transplantation may find itself at the forefront of the attack on never-say-die American medicine. The rise in transplantation, after cyclosporine was approved in 1983, happens to coincide with the United States health care explosion. In 1983, there were 164 liver transplants in the United States. Today, there are more than 3,000 per year. In 1984, surveys of the top problems facing the United States didn't even mention health care, an economic report from the Federal Reserve Bank of Dallas noted in 1993. Today, reform is perhaps the top priority of several state governments as well as the Clinton administration.

The numbers are shocking: Medical care prices have tripled since 1980. Hospital profits, or surpluses for nonprofits, have been rising steadily since 1988. And the Commerce Department says if expenditures continue to grow at the current rate, health care will represent a larger share of the United States gross domestic product than manufacturing by the year 2000. What consumed fifteen percent of the federal budget in 1992 will gobble twenty-eight percent by 2002, according to the

Congressional Budget Office. In 1990, the United States spent more than $666 billion on health care, almost double what Canada, Germany, Japan, Sweden, and the United Kingdom combined spent that year.

At the same time, occupancy in hospitals has been falling, to sixty-six percent by 1991 from seventy-six percent a decade earlier, according to an American Hospital Association survey. Since 1980, 1,000 hospitals have closed or merged.

The bottom line: Hospitals must find new ways to fill beds.

Transplantation plays a small but significant part in all of that. And transplant surgeons, hospital administrators, and others in the field have quickly realized that the numbers game they battle will not just be on the wall charts, but also in the legislatures.

With that in mind, Roger Evans, the health care finance researcher at the Mayo Clinic, tried to figure out how much profit is built into transplantation. It's not an easy task. "You can't get the numbers. Nobody really knows. The studies that have tried to take a guess say as much as fifty percent, but no one really knows," says Dr. Evans, a sociologist by training.

At Baylor, not even the financial experts dealing with patient bills know. Some doctors have "heard" that the not-for-profit—but nevertheless very wealthy—hospital makes a twenty to twenty-five percent profit on its billings for transplant care, below the Evans estimate. Others have heard the Baylor rate may be higher. Boone Powell, Jr., the hospital's president, will say only that the transplant program "makes money."

Consider only the liver transplant program at Baylor. The cost for a liver transplant generally runs around $150,000—about the national average for the simplest cases. Pittsburgh can run at least $300,000. How does it all add up so fast? As anyone who has spent time in a hospital knows, charges seem to multiply exponentially. Need a portable chest

■

X ray? One hundred dollars or so. Biopsy? There's the $36 biopsy-needle tray, the bill for the lab work, the $506 bill for the radiology if the biopsy has to be done with ultrasound, and then a bill for "interpreting" the results. Boom—$1,000. Every blood test runs up the tab, twice a day. Every pill taken costs something, every room is hundreds of bucks, every day in the ICU is thousands.

The average cost nationally of a liver transplant is now over $180,000, and some transplant patients have run up bills exceeding $1 million, even $4 million. At Baylor, $20,000 of the total tab comes from the transplant surgeons, who charge a flat fee for the surgery and all the follow-up and recovery—a fee patients say is the bargain of the year. The Southwest Organ Bank charges another $19,000 for recovery of the liver; various doctors such as the kidney specialists, radiologists, anesthesiologists, assisting surgeons, and others charge their fees—$50 to $150 every time they visit the patient's room, and a couple of thousand for O.R. services. Laboratories—inside and outside the hospital—bill for their services, and when all is said and done, the hospital's charge, another unbelievably thick bill, amounts to about two-thirds of the cost, or at least $100,000 for a simple two- or three-week stay.

Since the hospital performs about 150 transplants per year, Klintmalm's liver program brings in at least $15 million in gross revenue to Baylor, which has annual revenues of about $500 million per year. That doesn't count kidney transplants, heart and lung transplants, or even bone marrow transplants, nor does it include the benefits of boosting the hospital's reputation and competitive position by having one of the world's finest liver transplant programs. "We are better because we have it," Powell says. Fifteen million dollars is a significant sum for one program but not as dominant as in Pittsburgh, where transplantation of all kinds amounts to about thirty-five percent of the medical center's business.

No wonder then so many hospitals now want to enter the game. Liver transplantation is now at least a $500 million industry, a market growing so fast that hospitals have offered million-dollar signing bonuses to lure coveted transplant surgeons. Since 1988, the number of liver transplant programs in the United States has nearly doubled to 105 as hospitals have sought to build their technical reputations, boost billings, fill beds, generate media attention, keep local patients in town for treatment, and even lift staff morale. By pushing into transplantation, several hospital departments, such as pathology and radiology and anesthesiology, are challenged to improve their expertise. The "miracles" that soon take place at the hospital can be highly visible on the local evening news in the early days of a program. "It has a great halo effect," says Dr. James Thompson, chief of surgery at the University of Texas Medical Branch-Galveston, who launched a liver program in 1992.

"There's money to be made in liver transplantation— not many people running hospitals around the country aren't aware of that. People are trying to get organs because they are a valuable resource," says transplant surgeon Todd Howard at Washington University in St. Louis. "Transplantation right now is where trauma was ten or fifteen years ago. Every hospital wanted to be a trauma center before they found out it was expensive, and now they are trying to get out of it. A lot of hospitals see transplantation as helping to save their bottom line."

Consider what has happened in Texas. While Klintmalm built his program and reputation at Baylor, he had the state—and the whole Southwest—virtually all to himself. Houston's hospitals had renowned heart programs, with Cooley and DeBakey, but no liver efforts of substance. Then, when the boom really took off in the late 1980s and early 1990s, a program popped up in Houston, benefiting from the Houston organ bank's ability to control organs from Fort Worth. San Antonio, in the middle of the state, started a program, completing its first transplant in sixteen hours in 1992, when both Klintmalm and Goldstein were both routinely replacing a liver in four or five hours. Then Lubbock, a dusty west Texas college town, started a program. Its first liver transplant in 1993 lasted an even more daunting twenty hours, and the patient had to be retransplanted one week later.

Oklahoma, which used to send both patients and livers to Dallas, started a program at Oklahoma Memorial Hospital in Oklahoma City. Results were dismal: Five of the first fifteen patients were dead in less than a year. Soon a second program started nearby at Baptist Medical Center. New York City has two liver transplant programs. But Oklahoma City?

The second program—at Baptist Medical Center—is unique in its audacity, if not its ambition. It is the creation of Dr. Nazih Zuhdi, a wealthy, Lebanese-born cardiac surgeon hell-bent on establishing a liver capital to go with his successful heart program. In six months, Zuhdi, a friend of Dr. Christiaan Barnard, who made his fortune in medical device development in Minneapolis, says he spent "multi-millions," much of it from his own checkbook, to gather the liver talent. He brought in a Starzl-trained surgeon along with a renowned hepatologist, Dr. David Van Thiel, who in turn brought along a seventeen-person research squad and a computer expert.

Overnight, Baptist had to have an additional telephone operator. Operating rooms were remodeled, treatment rooms added on. Offices were reassigned and renovated, the prior occupants shunted to portable trailers in the parking lot. Plans were drawn for construction of a new transplant building, complete with garden suites and research facilities for Nobel Prize winners. "I always aim for the best," Zuhdi says.

Zuhdi predicts his program will do fifty liver transplants in its first full year and 100 the next. The livers will have to come from outside Oklahoma, since only about thirty are procured in the state annually, but they will be available, he says, if mediocre programs are closed, freeing more organs across regions.

"Before we decide which patient takes the organ, we should decide which center takes the organ," Zuhdi says. Others may have good programs, he says, "but not like the one I have." Solid patient-survival statistics over time will tell if he's right.

Another byproduct of this competition has been higher prices, which also flies in the face of conventional wisdom about free-market competition. In most marketplaces, so many suppliers chasing market share from a limited market would inevitably mean brutal price wars. Yet, despite the fact that the average hospital stay after a heart transplant is only a third as long as it was in 1984, the cost is twenty-five percent higher, even after adjusting for the medical rate of inflation. In another study of liver transplant costs, researchers found that hospitals that do more procedures, charge more per procedure, rather than less as might be expected under normal economic theory. What's more, the length of patient hospital stays in programs that did more transplants was actually shorter—and their bills were still bigger.

"It's a microcosm of some of the problems we face in health care," the Mayo Clinic's Dr. Evans says. "The charge should be substantially lower. Many of these [laws of economics] don't seem to apply well in medicine."

Insurance companies are trying to take the lead in reforming the system, negotiating discount contracts with transplant centers that have good success rates and lower costs, then establishing payment schedules to steer patients there. Medicare, too, designates centers now. "The insurers argue strongly that they can take the matter in their own hands, and it is consistent with the whole idea of managed care or preferred providers," Dr. Evans said.

At Baylor, one-third of the patients come through contracts with major insurance companies. The insurers offer patients only a handful of programs to pick from, sometimes calibrating benefits to make the decision more obvious. The

■

insurer might pay 100 percent of the cost in Birmingham, Alabama, for example, where a small, highly regarded program is well established and hospital costs are lower, but only seventy-five percent of the cost in Chicago.

At Baylor, Klintmalm offers seminars for insurers and courts good relations with the major firms. The more advanced the field becomes, the more challenges there are for the insurance companies, who have to decide if a treatment is worth paying for—if the chance of only thirty-percent success is worth $500,000, for example. Educating the insurers—marketing to them—is one way to smooth the system.

Transplant patients at Baylor must be preapproved by their insurance company before they are put on the waiting list, and that can take three or four weeks of review and haggling. There are no exceptions—even for a patient with rapidly spreading cancer, who could die because of that wait. Baylor asks for expedited reviews and approval from insurance companies, but that usually shaves only a week off the wait. Lack of strictness about financial clearance can lead to enormous headaches—and tragedy. The University of Pittsburgh faced a lawsuit after a heart patient was listed on the waiting list before financial clearance came. When a heart came up for the patient, it was used in a different man due to the lack of clearance. The waiting patient then died before another heart could be found.

The wording of insurance policies gets trickier and trickier, too, constantly changing to keep up with, or to outpace, the medical advances. Many policies now say they cover transplantation of "human organs"—an obvious exclusion of animal organs such as baboons or pigs. Many refer to "solid organs"—often leaving the question of coverage for bone marrow transplants for courts to decide.

Alison Victoria, the financial administrator, is the intermediary between the patient and the insurer. An artist by night and bureaucrat by day, she seems out of place around conservative Baylor with her orange hair and sometimes sharp views. For the patients, she is a strong advocate. For the hospital, she is a careful guardian of financial security. It is a job that borders sometimes on gut-wrenching nightmares. Alison wins most of her battles for patients but not all. "There are days when I say, 'Oh, please don't send me any more problems,' " she says. One day Randy Roady walked in unannounced with a puppy-dog face and two grocery sacks full of bills. He had a pocketful of checks from his insurance company, who was making payments to him instead of to the doctors and hospital. Randy asked if Alison could figure out who was supposed to get what. Two hours later, she had it all sorted and solved.

In recent years, the problems in transplantation have taken on renewed angst. The field has been under fire lately amid health care reform movements. While on the national stage, transplantation held its own in Hillary Rodham Clinton's efforts, it has been attacked at the state level as a high-technology procedure that society can do without, "given a utilitarian orientation towards doing the greatest good for the largest number of people," Dr. Evans noted in his examination of liver transplantation costs. The view is shared internationally, Evans said, pointing to a survey of seventy-five public health directors in England and Wales who were asked to rank in order of priority twelve treatments. Hip replacements ranked first; liver transplants eleventh, behind AIDS treatment and ahead only of advanced lung cancer treatment.

"Surveys such as this suggest that the future of liver transplantation may be imperiled," Evans concluded. But transplant surgeons and others shouldn't fear defending their programs. Cost-benefit analysis have shown that liver transplants compare quite favorably with other risky, expensive medical procedures. Saving a life and returning a person to work can have great economic benefit, and the field should be able to successfully defend itself, Evans says.

But there are other chinks in the armor. In 1993, Evans published a study in *The Journal of the American Medical Association* questioning the wide disparity in organ bank procurement charges. For livers, the most expensive organ, charges by the local organ bank ranged from $4,775 to $65,652 (in 1988 dollars), according to Evans's study. The median charge was $16,281 for a liver. That covers the bill at the donor's hospital—operating room for the harvest surgery and other charges—as well as the cost of the airplanes and ambulances, preservation fluids, fees to the transplant surgeons, and all the overhead of running the organ bank. Further, some hospitals were found to be marking up the organ bank charge when they passed it on to the patient. The Association of Organ Procurement Organizations reported in its latest annual report that organ banks' average charge to acquire a liver in 1991 was $13,791, suggesting that the hospital markup is significant.

Organ banks average about three organs out of each donor that can be placed in transplant patients. Sometimes they strike out if the organs turn out to be diseased; sometimes they hit a home run, placing the liver, two kidneys, the heart, the lungs, and the pancreas, a potential help to seven different patients awaiting organs. Either way, the flat charge is made for each organ. Organ banks also can recover costs by using bone, tissue, corneas, and other parts for transplantation. Given the actual cost of hospital operating rooms, Lear jets, and other services, as well as the fees paid to surgeons for the donor surgery, Evans found the organ bank charges to be high. And while there was still debate over whether the families should receive some financial incentive or reward for donating, he concluded that the not-for-profit organ banks themselves were benefiting from lucrative financial incentives. Yet, since organ donation rates have declined for the past three years, possibly as the result of seatbelt laws, airbags, and changes in society, or possibly the result of inefficiency on the part of the organ banks, one might

■

215

also suggest that the lure of financial incentives doesn't seem to work in organ donation. Said Evans:

> "Based on the data presented herein, it is clear that 'the gift of life' can be financially lucrative to hospitals and OPOs [Organ Procurement Organizations, or organ banks].... Cost-effectiveness is threatened when per-procedure expenditures increase and benefits remain unchanged. Thus, even if more lives are saved due to increased organ donation, the relative cost-effectiveness of transplantation will deteriorate. This, in turn, makes transplantation vulnerable to the public health challenge associated with controlling health care expenditures. It would seem the transplant community would do well to become more fiscally responsible than it is today."

The response from the organ banks? "Transplantation is no more lucrative than eye surgery or taking care of pregnant women. Medicine is a lucrative business," Dr. James Burdick, chairman of the United Network for Organ Sharing ethics committee, replied on the front page of *USA Today*, where Roger Evans's study was the lead story.

Concerned about the rising costs, Bob Goldstein once ordered the air-charter company working for the Southwest Organ Bank to stop supplying plates of fresh seafood and champagne for meals on flights. Instead, the pilots are usually asked to find some omelets at Denny's while the surgeons are off at the hospital, and the pilots always keep a cooler of soft drinks and Beck's beer on board the airplanes. A beer for the doctors on the way home with the liver is traditional and soothing. Other surgeons tell stories of transplant surgeons arriving for a harvest in limousines. Ambulances, needed for the race of heart retrievals but really not necessary for liver harvests, are still used out of tradition, even though they are expensive. But in some cities, the Baylor team simply takes a cab to the local hospital to hold down costs—and bad impressions. (Patients, though, might cringe to think of their livers in the greasy trunk of the rickety cab that often greets the team in Lubbock and the one-handed cowboy cab driver with a long, scraggly beard and leather duster who tries to amuse surgeons with jokes about the body parts he has shuttled.)

Yet another issue for a public wringing its hands over health care may be the income doctors are making. It can be a delicate subject. Tom Starzl fumes when he begins reciting the list of disciples who have cashed in on his creation, moved into mansions, and taken up expensive hobbies such as racing fancy sports cars. Starzl draws a salary as a University of Pittsburgh medical professor of more than $200,000. He lives well, but modestly. He is probably one of the lowest paid heads of a transplant program in the country, and, when he was operating, one of the lowest paid transplant surgeons. He believes, rather naively, that those he trained should commit their careers to research and to saving lives and that flaunting fancy lifestyles will only undermine public perceptions and hurt the field.

Perhaps. But transplant surgeons have a special skill and make a remarkable contribution to society. Their millions may not be out of line with brain surgeons or fancy orthopedic surgeons or highbrow plastic surgeons or even big-time lawyers and corporate chairmen who can cash in on million-dollar stock options and six- and seven-figure salaries. The earnings of transplant surgeons are certainly comparable to those of backup quarterbacks or mediocre relief pitchers and probably amount to far less than the salaries of twenty-two-year-old rookie basketball players who happen to be seven-feet tall, all of which may say something quite profound about what's important in our society. No one dies if Shaquille O'Neil has a bad night.

In any event, transplant surgery can be a lucrative profession—if you are good at it. For Goran Klintmalm, building his program into the powerhouse that it has become has landed him in the social circles of the elite. He has a good deal with Baylor because he does well for the hospital. Most of his staff in his Transplant Services offices—the secretaries and coordinators and dietitians and computer specialists—are paid by the hospital. Money for research nurses often comes from drug companies and other grants. There are numerous other expenses, such as salaries of $30,000 per year or so for the surgical fellows and miscellaneous office expenses, but a large pot of money is still left over for the partnership of Klintmalm, Goldstein, and Husberg to share. (Marlon Levy earned a salary for two years before he becomes a partner in 1994.) How big is the pot? Just from liver transplants, the partnership bills about $3 million per year. What is collected is lower, of course. Collections typically run sixty to eighty percent. That means revenue of something around $2 million before fees for the sixty kidney transplants the team does each year and before fees the team collects from the organ bank for its harvest surgery. Office expenses, including malpractice insurance premiums, can eat half of that income, according to a study of transplant programs. So the partners probably have something more than $1 million to split.

To most patients, grateful for the second chance at life, that is exactly the way it should be—the surgeons should be rewarded for their hard work, skill, and even their pain and suffering in such a grueling profession. They are forced to take huge risks and make tough choices, and their fees are far easier for patients to accept then the far higher charges of the hospital and even of the laboratories, which can charge between $200 and $300 every time a blood sample is drawn and a drug

■

level is checked, or $1,000 a month for life-sustaining drugs such as cyclosporine. This is the American way after all—those who achieve are rewarded for their success. It is one of the reasons Klintmalm left Sweden—those who achieve there are not rewarded any more than the dolts, he says.

Yet all doctors are under fire in the health care reform environment, and those at the top, such as transplant surgeons, may attract some sharp incoming missiles because hospitals turn away patients who can't afford the expensive procedure. Klintmalm's partnership often tries to work with patients in financial straits, agreeing to accept an insurance company's payment even if it is less than the standard charge, as they did for Randy Roady, or offering a discount for a cash-paying customer such as Arden Lynn trying to survive on a dwindling nest egg. The hospital and other doctors do the same. And yet patients are still turned away because of the high cost, companies still lay off employees because their health coverage premiums are escalating (General Motors says $929 of the cost of every car it makes goes to health care for employees), and taxpayers are still asked to cough up more because of rising medical expenditures.

These are hard questions for our society to face. Still, one might argue that in his neck of the woods, Goran Klintmalm is far more valuable than Manny Lee, a backup shortstop for the Texas Rangers who made more money in 1993 and stepped up to the plate fewer times than Klintmalm stood at the operating room table. And beyond Tom Starzl, one might also have to wonder how quickly the field would have developed, and how rapidly the treatment been made available to people, if there were not rich financial rewards on the table.

How to pay for liver transplants may well become a bigger issue than who should do them, or when they should be done, or who should receive them. Somehow the nation must find a way to continue to advance health care, to take advantage of our talents, to resist the temptation to slide back, per-

■

haps with arbitrary rules to limit access, or short-sighted restrictions on rewards. And yet somehow we must also find a way to avoid bankrupting ourselves. Once again, transplantation mirrors the entire national health care situation. Just as we are on the verge of major breakthroughs in this science of saving lives, so too may we be also on the verge of major changes in how we save lives, and when we save them, and which lives we save. And how we pay for it.

CHAPTER 12

THE CURSE
OF ROTTEN TIMING

S he had been on the waiting list since August, and now it was January. Arden Lynn, who had been called in as a backup and lost out to the younger woman in a coma, was counting each day, and slipping each day as well. "You really want the sickest to go first, it's a heartfelt feeling," she said. Yolanda Contreras, after more than thirty days of being locked in a coma after receiving the liver Lynn might have had, had woken up, moved to the fourteenth floor for recovery and then to Twice Blessed House. That comforted Arden. But now, she was sure she had to be among the sickest. She worried that her luck, however, had run out.

So much had happened since that startling October day when she waited by the elevators caught up in life-and-death emotions. She had closed out the estates of her father and her husband. She had spent many hours trying to take care of her own medical bills—a stress she was sure other patients, who had insurance, did not wrestle with as constantly as she did. With Alison Victoria, she battled Social Security for disability, and cursed the insurance company that canceled her policy after her Warren shunt surgery that rerouted blood flow to the liver in order to relieve stress on the crippled organ. How could the insurance company do that? It was tragic, she thought in retrospect. It had taken her four years to find a company that would offer her any kind of policy, and then only one that cov-

■

221

ered her up to $50,000. Around the transplant unit, $50,000 is only a fraction of the down payment. And she was too young for Medicare—sixty, instead of sixty-two. Along with everything else, Arden Lynn had lousy timing.

More than anything else, Arden Lynn felt abandoned by the system, a victim who had done nothing wrong. She had lived a middle class life, and now she was suddenly nearly too poor to support herself. And there was little help. Nobody at the agencies returned her phone calls. Nobody gave any hope of assistance. Her money was running out, and as the weeks stretched on, four weeks after the backup call, then eight, ten, now twelve, the meter was ticking away. Halloween turned into Thanksgiving, Christmas into New Year's. Her daughter was so stressed she was covered with hives. "Bill [Arden's husband] died a year ago today," Arden said in late December, after seventeen weeks on the waiting list. "And Dad died on the twenty-first. It's a bad season for us."

Through the fall and winter, Arden followed every high and low of the transplant team via the Bryans and other friends she had picked up around Baylor, keeping special tabs on Mrs. Contreras, for whom she now felt a special kind of battlefield brotherhood. She was relieved that Don Bryan was improving, having worried that he, like she, had waited too long and might not be able to recover. And she had been fascinated by Tom Starzl's baboon liver attempt, especially since she had come to believe that the waiting list was her worst enemy, and any advance that might ease the waiting list woes was vital. She worried over whether to enter the special study of FK 506 offered to her, reluctant to take an "experimental" medicine but equally worried about passing up any advantage. It made a huge financial difference to Lynn as well. Cyclosporine could cost up to $1,000 per month; FK 506 was free until approved beyond experimental status.

And more than anything, she wondered how long a wait was too long, for she was convinced there was such a point. "Is

■

there a precipice I'll go over?" she asked, knowing the answer was "yes," having seen Contreras almost fall too far herself. Arden stopped getting dressed up for her appointments with Dan Polter and stopped wearing makeup, fearing that she was making too good, too healthy, an impression at the hospital. No sense in not looking as sick as she really was at this point. "I don't think I can sit around and do nothing but wait much longer," she said one day. "I need someone to step in front of a bus." To Polter she had put in an order: She would like any liver, but she would prefer a fifteen-year-old Mormon liver.

One night Arden had been unable to sleep and was listening to one of those all-night radio call-in shows to pacify her anxiety. With typical sensitivity, the host was making fun of the baboon liver recipient in Pittsburgh, telling "jokes" about the guy "swinging from the chandelier." And then he got to the crux of his show, wondering whether these crazy transplants, baboon or human, are worthwhile at all. "Why do this?" he wondered.

At 3:15 A.M., Arden had heard enough. She called in, got on the air, and told her story—how transplants offered the only hope for lots of different diseases, how people were dying on the waiting list because there were not enough organs to go around, how research such as the baboon liver experiment might solve that problem, and how she might very well be one of the ones who died waiting. "That shut him up and all the others," she said. "He said, 'I didn't realize.' "

"I've never done anything like that in my life," Arden said, half wondering what had gotten into her, and yet fully knowing that it was an outburst of her own frustration.

The call from Baylor finally came just after midnight, 144 days after she first got her beeper and almost twelve weeks after that October day when she wondered if she would ever get another chance. She had already taken her antianxiety medication, Xanax, when she answered the phone, so she stayed calm. "The minute the phone rang, I knew what it was," she said. In

October, she had been laughing and crying, but this time, Arden was a cool professional. She woke up her daughter, who rushed over, and decided to let her son sleep. At six A.M., she called him from the hospital, and he was there in "oh, about a minute and a half."

The surgery began at eight A.M., with Klintmalm and Distant at the controls.

Lars Backman and Bob Goldstein had gone overnight to Tyler, a nearby Texas town, to retrieve the liver. It was a horrible trip, not that any are all that delightful. After a while, all the surgeons harden themselves to the tragedies of the donors, almost all of whom die suddenly, and tragically, and often horribly. This one was among the worst: a fifteen-year-old suicide victim. To make matters worse, the winter weather was lousy. The plane couldn't land in Tyler, which is only about an hour's drive away anyway, so they circled, then landed "somewhere, who knows where," Backman recalled, then took a one-hour ambulance ride. Goldstein slept on the stretcher the whole way.

In Dallas, Klintmalm wanted to do the surgery himself because undoing the Warren shunt would be a little tricky. But he was nothing but smooth and swift that morning. GK and Dale had Arden out of the O.R. in rapid order, finishing with no complications despite the complexity. She went to the intensive care unit and woke up quickly.

"Well, I got you a fifteen-year-old liver," a beaming Dan Polter told her. "I don't know if it was Mormon or not, but it is fifteen years old."

Arden just smiled, making rapid progress. On the second day, she startled Bo Husberg during rounds.

"Husberg walked in and I said, 'Well, how are you?'"

"He said, 'What did you say?!'"

"'How are you?'"

"'No patient has ever asked me that in the ICU,' he said. 'I guess you are doing very well.'"

■

"Somebody has to look out for these doctors," Arden quipped.

So impressed was Husberg that he moved Arden to the fourteenth floor that day, an abbreviated ICU stay that delighted her as both economical and hopeful. "I'm so excited," she said once on the transplant floor. "I'm so anxious to get better."

Arden had waited so long that the contract for the FK 506 dosing study had expired, and Klintmalm and the pharmaceutical company, Fujisawa, were at odds over some of the details of who could control dosage in further trials. Klintmalm wanted total control since they were his patients. Fujisawa wanted to put in some guarantees that it would get the data it needed for the study, which was designed to find the optimal dose of the drug by giving some patients high doses, some low doses, and finding the best starting point somewhere in the middle. The issue was whether a patient Klintmalm thought might be in danger and need a different dose would have to stick to the dose prescribed by the study for a brief time. It was a battle Klintmalm eventually won, but in the interim, no new patients were added to the study. So in that brief early January period, Arden Lynn and others didn't have a choice, they had to stick to tried-and-true cyclosporine. To Arden, it was no matter. She was on her way to an easy recovery.

Or so she thought. By Day Three, her bilirubin had doubled, from 3.0 to 6.0. Her other numbers on the almost virgin wall chart were rising faster than a bull market. Husberg ordered a liver biopsy, ASAP.

In the pathology lab, there was no debate. "Acute cellular rejection" was the diagnosis. Arden had had her new liver less than seventy-two hours, and already her body was violently rejecting it. Her hopes sank as low as her numbers soared: bilirubin up to 7.0, then 12, then 13. A recycle of steroids was started—feeding her megadoses even though she was already still on some very high doses because it had only been a few days since the surgery. Now, when the team walked into the

■

room, there was no need to look at the wall chart to get an idea of how the patient was doing. Arden Lynn, lying in bed, was bright yellow.

"You're doing OK," Klintmalm tried to reassure her. It was faint praise. Concern was growing because the rejection had set in so fast and so strong. Arden's daughter was nervous, her son so worried that Tom Renard took him aside to calm him down.

One waiting game had been replaced by another. There was really nothing the team could do but wait to see if the steroids would work. If not, then OKT-3 would be the next weapon. If that didn't work, maybe she could be converted to FK. If that didn't work, it was back on the list for another liver. There were a lot of possibilities, none of them particularly enticing.

And there was this question: Would any of this have happened if she had been on FK, which was thought to be a bit better at preventing rejection, instead of cyclosporine? Was her timing so bad, missing out on the FK 506 study, that it might, indeed, kill her?

One week out, Arden's numbers were still up, and GK was talking about OKT-3. He would come by three times a day to check on her. And by that afternoon, things began to turn, or so it seemed. Her bilirubin was back down to 7.0. "You're doing MUCH better!" Klintmalm extolled, and Arden clapped.

"Can I take a shower tomorrow?" she joked, hardly able to sit up in bed, let alone get out of it.

"Yes, we don't want you too grungy," Klintmalm chuckled, turning to the team and ordering that the intravenous line started in anticipation of the OKT-3 therapy be taken out. The danger was passing, but there would be another biopsy Friday.

Like any good roller coaster, the results were not what anyone expected. Arden was still rejecting according to the biopsy, even though her numbers were slowly coming down. Facing the diagnosis of residual rejection, knowing that the numbers lag as an indicator and may turn soon, Klintmalm ordered OKT-3—the magic bullet, the miracle monoclonal antibody you can only take once in your life (over a two-week course of doses).

OKT-3—sometimes referred to in the hallways as Okey-Dokey and Shake and Bake—is designed to destroy the killer cells attacking the liver, but the danger is it can assassinate much more. It can attack the heart muscle and cause cardiac arrest, for example. Once, doctors at the Hoag Heart Institute in Newport Beach, Calif., were running low on their usual immunosuppressant medication, Atgam, so they gave a few heart transplant patients this new OKT-3 for routine prevention of rejection. It was the first time the hospital had ever used OKT-3. Four patients died, according to a government report. The hospital explained it this way in a statement for the report: "Unfortunately, the drug proved to be too powerful for immunosuppression."

Before OKT-3 was given, Arden had to have a chest X ray, an EKG test of her heart, and a slew of other assays. A cardiac resuscitation cart was wheeled to the ready. Monitors were hooked up. One of the fellows had to sit by the bedside for the first hour after the drug was administered, alert to fire up the cardiac resuscitation paddles if need be. It was one of the few times that the patient's tension is matched by that of the doctors and nurses. Everyone is on edge around OKT-3. And for the patients, there is a cruel irony: The better the drug works, the sicker it makes you.

Saturday afternoon, Arden was not handling the drug well at all. She was getting sicker and sicker, beyond the point where it seems the drug is simply working well. Arden was slipping further and further, looking to nurses and doctors alike that this might well be BIG TROUBLE. Her heart got a bit erratic. Her nausea escalated. She was rushed back downstairs to the intensive care unit within an hour of her first OKT-3 dose, but only got worse. By nightfall, her heartbeat was irregular. She had gone into atrial fibrillation ("a-fib" in hospital slang), which means her heart was completely erratic and might well just quit on any beat. Robert, her son, paced the hallway. That night, he was told, she would either live or die, either turn the corner or not make it. At one point, he was told the next hour could decide it all. Tom Renard stood at her bedside monitoring her minute by minute, heartbeat by heartbeat. "They thought they'd lose her for a while," said Robert, scared and stressed. Indeed, the team thought Arden Lynn might very well be dead in the next hour.

Arden survived that hour, and the next, and the next. By Monday, she was still having heart troubles, but that was treatable, she and Robert were told. The OKT-3 appeared to be working on the rejection, even though she was a wreck, sleeping only ten minutes at a time, wondering why such a fate had befallen her. "It was all very scary," she said of the weekend, trying to force a smile in her ICU bed. "If I had known it was going to be this much fun, I'd tell everyone to get one."

Robert asked Bob Goldstein if the problem was with the liver that she got. No, the liver was OK, it was her body that was trying to kill it, Goldstein explained. At the bedside, a resident pointed out that two cultures had come back positive for infection, so an antibiotic was added to the brew of medications she was receiving. Infection—another worry. They go hand in hand, infection and rejection. To kill the rejection, you have to disable the body's own immune system. But doing that can let infections run rampant. Statistically, those that get infections usually have had rejection episodes.

Goldstein had earlier tried to give Arden that day's dose of OKT-3. But as she was premedicated—treated for the nausea and other side effects—she went into atrial fibrillation again. "We'll try later," he said. "She has to get the dose."

Some choice: If she gets it, she may die; if she doesn't, she'll surely die.

"Be aggressive about her low potassium," Goldstein

■

told the fellows. "I'm worried about a heart attack." Low potassium can lead to heart attacks. Arden had been retaining fluid, so she was on high doses of diuretics to flush out extra fluid. With the fluid often goes the potassium. Everything seemed connected somehow to everything else.

In addition, she wasn't eating, and nutrition was a concern. A feeding tube would be necessary tomorrow if she couldn't eat, Goldstein said.

After all that, he turned to Arden, smiled and said, "Everything looks good."

She mustered a sarcastic "I'm glad you think so," and sighed, confiding later that she was well aware of her predicament, and understandably terrified. "I just wish it would go away," she said. "It"—all the trouble, all the heartache, all the waiting, all the fighting. Why couldn't "it" just go away?

Yet "it" got even worse. Arden's white blood cell count almost fell to zero—0.4 actually, off the charts and almost into oblivion. Her temperature spiked to 105 degrees, and nobody knew why. She was placed in isolation in the ICU unit and given massive doses of drugs, such as a biotech breakthrough called Neupogen, to build her count back up. It was yet another complication that could kill her, yet another one she beat. Slowly, the white count came back. And by February, Arden was moved back up to the fourteenth floor. What she had hoped would be a speedy and affordable recovery had turned into a physical and financial nightmare.

Getting back up to the room wasn't much comfort. A young girl in the room next door, who had gone into rejection because she had stopped taking her immunosuppressive drugs at home, spiraled down each hour and died in the middle of one night—a terrible episode for all who had known her on the floor, compounded by a mother crying hysterically at the nurses' station. Arden now had to contend with massive pain in her arm from an infection, probably from one of the many IV lines running there. If drugs didn't clear it up, she might have to have a vein surgically removed, she was told. Her feet were swollen, her numbers actually climbing a bit. The bilirubin was back over 3.0. "All I can see is money going up, up, up, up," she said. "I had no idea it would be like this. Tell me something is going good. *Something* must be going good. I need some encouragement."

CHAPTER 13
THE CUTTING EDGE

Lars Backman was losing the patient. Blood pressure was dropping, blood was pouring over the sides of the abdomen onto the operating room floor. Backman, his magnifying loupes on, was frantically searching for the source of the bleeding, a probe in one hand, an argon coagulator in the other to burn close the hidden wound.

It had been a relatively normal transplant operation for the Swedish fellow. Backman had opened the abdomen and cut off most all the connections to the liver as usual. The operating room had become a little tense when the patient began to bleed through a hole in the portal vein, but Backman had closed it quickly with little drop in blood pressure. Music was on the radio, chatter swirled above the open belly . . . Madonna's underwear, stuff like that. All was normal until the patient began bleeding uncontrollably from some hidden wound. Backman and the others had no idea what the problem was.

Was it the spot where he sewed together the vena cava? One stitch too deep and maybe he caught the back wall, pulling it closed and cutting off the blood flow, forcing a rupture upstream. Maybe the liver had no way to drain blood and had exploded open on the underside? Or maybe the source of trouble was a stitch that merely skimmed the tissue, like a fish hook that doesn't catch deep enough in the prey, letting the trophy bass escape by pulling free? Backman frantically lifted up

■

the liver trying to find something underneath that would lead him to the answer before it was too late.

Maybe over there, an assisting surgeon kept suggesting impetuously. Anesthesiologists were desperately pumping blood into the patient, trying to maintain pressure high enough for life. Blood was carried in by the bucket not the bag, and the latest came into the operating room with a warning: This was all there was, for now.

"Shit!" Backman bellowed politely, but nervously. "Could you please hold this back for me?"

The bleeding continued. The patient's heart, exposed to the ceiling and measurable without any fancy monitors or graphs, slowed and slowed, like the last gasps of a deflating balloon. Numbers were called out, but there really was no need. Everyone in the room could see the feeble heart, which seemed to be having a hard time deciding if this would be the last beat, or maybe the next beat would be the last. The numbers kept going down. And down. The only thing going up was frustration.

Backman was losing the battle. Maybe this was all the result of some rare reaction to transfused blood. Resignation spread through the room. This one just wasn't going to make it.

It happens.

"The spleen!" he called out. "Maybe it's the spleen?"

Three people—six hands—all dove for the sack of blood inside the body that stores reserves to be released when an extra spurt of blood is needed. Maybe it had ruptured or been cut? When you bleed from the spleen, you bleed big time, and this patient was just about big time bled out. The spleen was a good guess.

One surgeon grabbed it, another pulled back intestines and organs and Backman tied it off and cut it out, all in a matter of a minute or less. Sure enough, the six-inch-long bag had ruptured. An inch-long hole right in the middle had let pints

■

and pints of blood escape. The bleeding was stopped. Slowly but immediately, blood pressure bottomed out and then started to rise. The pace of the heartbeats began to speed up. The river of blood over the sides of the abdomen slowed to a stream, then a trickle.

The patient appeared to be saved.

"Let's let the pig stabilize for thirty minutes or so now," Backman said, relief etched on his brow.

On the operating room table was pig number 725, nicknamed Spot. He was part of a major research project at Baylor to try to determine what happens to blood inside the liver. Little is known, actually, about the dynamics of blood flow in the liver. Baylor's research chief, Dr. William Paulsen, and the transplant team developed a method to completely isolate the liver in a pig through transplant-like surgery. Then they are able to play with the liver without worrying about the effects from other organs. What happens if we do this? Or that? What parts of the transplant procedures are harmful to the liver? Beneficial? How can we improve, or at least cut down on the damage that occurs when the organ is moved from one body to the next? What drugs help, or hurt? What techniques are best? And is there a new way of thinking about the liver that would make transplanting easier?

Pig Number 725—Spot—almost didn't make it to the research phase of the project. Because of the bleeding, he almost died before the liver was completely isolated, before the experiment could begin.

The research goes on in a basically unmarked building near Roberts Hospital. Baylor buys farm pigs for about $80 apiece at the slaughterhouse auction, just like any bacon manufacturer. The pigs are kept in cages by veterinarians until the surgery. They are anesthetized and never allowed to wake up. For each experiment, two pigs are required: one for the actual surgery, and one to supply blood for the procedure. Thus when the bucket of blood came into the operating room for Spot, that was the last of what had been taken from another pig put to sleep for the same experiment.

Pigs have proved to be far better research animals than dogs, which were the original animal of transplant-experiment preference. "Pound dogs" often came with diseases or abnormalities that could affect the data. And because of the animal-rights outcry, they became much more politically incorrect—and harder to get. The last thing Baylor wanted was pickets outside its research lab and operating rooms.

"Besides," Backman said in his deep, serious voice, "the dogs often did not have insurance."

What pigs had over dogs most of all, besides health-insurance jokes, was an amazingly human-like liver. As any high school biology class dissector knows, pig anatomy is similar to humans—the reason why high schools use fetal pigs for science experiments. In the case of the liver, the similarities are so great that many in transplantation believe the day will come when pig livers are used instead of human livers. Representatives of one major hospital supply company have even told doctors that they have begun scouting pig farms in Iowa to get a jump on the competition and be the first to market with pig livers for human transplants.

In Los Angeles, Dr. Leonard Makowka, another Starzl protege, used a pig liver to try to save a dying twenty-six-year-old woman waiting for a liver. Susan Fowler's liver had failed completely, and a donor liver did not come available even though she was listed as "Status 4"—nationwide emergency priority—just like Rex Voss. So Makowka routed her blood through a pig liver transplanted into her abdomen. The woman lived off the pig-liver bridge for a day. Some called the move heroic, others called it reckless. Either way, it ultimately didn't work. Susan Fowler died before a human liver could be found and transplanted. The case not only punctuated the waiting-list crisis at the large transplant centers, but also tweaked curiosity for the potential of pig livers. It seemed to raise more questions than it answered. And it left the question of viability of "xenografting"—transplanting between species—perhaps even more a mystery than before the experiment.

At about the same time in the last half of 1992, none other than Tom Starzl dove into the headlines again with another first: a baboon-liver transplant. It had to be Starzl. Even three decades into transplantation, no one stretches and innovates and hunts for breakthroughs the way Starzl does. He had won permission from Pittsburgh's medical-ethics board for four baboon-liver transplants. It had never been done before— Starzl had tried putting baboon kidneys into humans almost thirty years earlier. Now was the time for baboon livers, he reasoned. Baboons were closer on the evolutionary chain to humans, so there might be fewer complications than with a pig liver. The way to do it, Starzl said, was to start as close to humans as you could and then work your way back to pigs as you learn more. He called the same baboon-breeding lab in San Antonio that had supplied him before with animals bred in captivity for research and placed his order.

Pittsburgh no longer offered human liver transplants to victims of hepatitis B—it always comes back, often destroying the transplanted liver. Dallas and others still transplant for hepatitis B, but Starzl had decided it was not the best use of such a limited resource. Human livers had to be saved for those with a better chance of survival. It was a bold position for a man who himself had the hepatitis B virus. Years before, Starzl developed hepatitis B from coming into contact with a patient's blood during surgery, and it almost killed him. Given the policy, hepatitis B patients were the perfect choice for his baboon-transplant attempts. They were people who, under his policy, had no other hope for a transplant. Starzl and others believed that the baboon might not be susceptible to recurrence of the

hepatitis B virus, that the animal liver was somehow protect-
ed. Armed with permission from the Institutional Review
Board, all Tom Starzl needed was a volunteer.

In the summer of 1992, Starzl's top three surgeons, a
jovial Greek named Andreas Tzakis, a skilled Japanese surgeon
named Satoru Todo, and a brilliant Chinese-American doctor
named John Fung, removed the liver from a baboon in one
operating room and carried it next door to transplant it into a
thirty-two-year-old patient who carried the deadly hepatitis
virus. The man's name was kept confidential, and the
announcement of the successful surgery set off headlines
around the world.

That day, animal-rights protesters began picketing outside Presbyterian Hospital, which is carved into the steep hill-
side on the University of Pittsburgh campus, adjacent to Pitt's
bowl-shaped football stadium at the crest of the hill. How could
you sacrifice one animal for human convenience, they asked?
Who gave them the right to destroy a baboon? It was an old
fight in medicine, rekindled.

Transplant patients, those waiting and those recovering, went out to face the protesters the next day. If they were
dying, they would see things differently, the patients said. If it
was their child, and there was no other hope, wouldn't it be different? There were not enough human livers, why weren't they
worried about that problem? The face-to-face drama was
compelling, and the protests died out in a few days, just as the
television cameras and live CNN broadcasts of Tzakis's news
conferences faded after only a few days.

The baboon liver functioned well, Tzakis reported. But
after several weeks the man developed a fungal infection—
aspergillosis—a simple mold coughed up by most people with
no harm. But in an immunosuppressed patient, aspergillis is
an opportunistic, deadly killer. In most cases, Tzakis said, what
spawns the fungus infection is too much suppression of the

immune system, and in this case, Starzl blamed high doses of a drug, Cytoxan, as part of the immunosuppressive cocktail. In a sense, it was the surgeons' missteps that allowed the aspergillis to take root. "The problem," Tzakis said later while strolling the corridors of the Pittsburgh complex, "is that by the time you realize there is too much immunosuppression, it is too late."

The only treatment for aspergillosis is an old antifungal drug called amphotericin B, so toxic that it can be taken only in small doses. A newer version, liposomal amphotericin B, is available in Europe and elsewhere in the world but not in the United States. The U.S. Food and Drug Administration is still studying it, weighing its steps oh so carefully. Liposomal amphotericin B is really the same drug delivered differently—attached to lipids, or fats, that help the drug penetrate to where it's needed without harsh side effects. More of the drug can be delivered, improving effectiveness.

Goran Klintmalm got to use liposomal amphotericin B once, for a thirty-four-year-old psychologist named Pam Blumenthal who had received a liver, kidney, and pancreas. Her family had been able to pressure the FDA into letting Klintmalm try liposomal amphotericin B on a compassionate basis. A cancer researcher in Houston was making the drug in his laboratory for research, and the FDA allowed him to manufacture some batches for Pam after senators from Texas and North Carolina, along with the White House, called the bureaucrat in the FDA who could release the drug. But it was too late. And three years later, neither Klintmalm nor Starzl nor anyone else had access to liposomal amphotericin B. "It is a crime that we still cannot get it," Klintmalm would fume when the subject, and the FDA, came up.

Regular amphotericin B did no good for Starzl's baboon-liver recipient, and he died on the seventieth day after transplant, ten weeks exactly. The next day, a secret was revealed:

■

The man had also had the HIV virus. Facing AIDS, he had basically offered his body to science. The disclosure raised even more questions about the ethics of medical experimentation.

Undeterred, Starzl tried again. The baboon liver, after all, had worked well and was still working the day the man died. The research would go on. This time, the patient was a sixty-two-year-old man, also unidentified, who also was dying of hepatitis B.

Andy Tzakis had done the surgery again, on a Sunday. Monday brought a news conference, Tuesday morning another appearance on the "Today" show. He had become something of a media star. Tzakis had come to Pittsburgh a decade earlier and actually was dispatched to Dallas in the early days of the program there to help Klintmalm. For a while, it was only the two of them, Klintmalm and Tzakis. And it proved to be the turning point in his career, giving Tzakis the skills and confidence to turn into one of the finest transplanters in the world. After he had transplanted, in 1990, a second liver into a young Texas girl named Stormie Jones, the first person to ever receive a heart and a liver, he appeared on CNN, and the broadcast was carried back home in Greece. His father, old and ill, got to see his son on television before he died. It was a very proud moment for Andy. Now, he was a star again. As he walked through the halls, he was tired from lack of sleep, but exhilarated with the experiment, and people stopped him in every corridor: "Saw you on the 'Today' show, Andy . . ."

At Pittsburgh, transplant patients are scattered all over the sprawling hospital complex, some at Presbyterian, some at Children's, some even at the Veterans Administration hospital. At Presbyterian, four floors of intensive care beds are devoted to transplant patients. The place is a miniature United Nations, holding patients of all nationalities who have come to the mecca of transplanting. Surgeons, too, have come from all over to train at the side of the master. Pittsburgh is the only place with a successful small-bowel transplant program, the only place to do a five-organ cluster transplant, the only place to do "xenografts." It has the air of chaos—no one seems to be in charge, but everything gets done, and done well. Underneath the seeming confusion is a solid organization. There is not one team but specialized entities each responsible for a specific ward, or a specific organ, or a specific part of the transplant surgery.

Patients too sick or too difficult for other centers end up in Pittsburgh—hundreds each year. They end up waiting longer than patients at other centers. Still, Pittsburgh has a one-year survival rate for livers above eighty percent—better than the national average, even though they do the most difficult cases by far.

"How is he today?" Tzakis asked a fellow as he approached the room, a cubicle with a sliding-glass door filled with pumps and monitors and one sixty-two-year-old baboon-liver recipient only a couple of days out of surgery.

"This baboon liver looked better than the last," Tzakis said, then turned to his fellow. "Dr. Starzl says stop the Cytoxan. Now. We will not give any more Cytoxan. You got it?"

Along with the liver, the patient received an injection of bone-marrow cells from the baboon as well. The bone-marrow transplant amounts to an infusion of genetic material, DNA, that Starzl now believes helps the recipient's body to accept the new organ. It is a crude form of genetic engineering, trying to trick the body into believing that the DNA in the transplanted liver is actually A-OK because it matches genetic material already in the immune system. One of the more interesting findings in the first baboon-liver transplant was that baboon DNA appeared later in the lungs of the man, indicating that there had been sharing of the genetic codes across the species.

Starzl calls it "chimerism," and he has now found the same phenomenon in some of his early human-human transplant patients as well. Genetic material from the donor, brought in through the transplanted liver, takes root in the

■

recipient's body, Starzl has found. The result is a third breed of DNA—a mix of the donor and recipient. It can seem like spooky stuff, taking on the genetic makeup of another, unrelated human, or even altering genetic makeup halfway through life. Yet the result is breath-taking: Some of Starzl's patients have actually stopped taking all their immunosuppressive drugs because their bodies have, through chimerism, accepted the foreign organ as genetically compatible. "We now suggest that most liver recipients who have an untroubled convalescence and survive more than five years have their drugs weaned under supervision, and stopped," Starzl said in a paper.

The finding shows when you get a liver, you really do get much more. Starzl's bone marrow technique offered hope not just for xenografts, but for routine liver transplants as well. If everyone got DNA from their donor through a bone marrow transplant, then the transplanted liver might be more acceptable to the patient's body, and the risk of rejection might be diminished. If that were true, doctors could get by with lower doses of immunosuppressive drugs, and the risk of infection or viruses might also be reduced.

Andy Tzakis donned a mask to keep the room as sterile as possible, and went in to see his famous, but anonymous, patient, who was now completely oblivious to the exciting research that he was a part of. "Richard. Richard. RICHARD!" Tzakis yelled, but the man slept. Andy slapped him across the face gently. "Richard wake up!"

"He's been like this all day," the resident reported with a shrug. "We've cut back on his sedation, but he still is not alert at all."

"Everything else is OK. Make sure he gets no more Cytoxan. Dr. Starzl said no more," Tzakis said, and turned to leave.

The sixty-two-year-old patient never did become very alert, and he died twenty-six days after his operation. A massive septic infection—peritonitis—had grown in his abdomen, killing him on February 5, 1993.

The next day, the Physicians Committee for Responsible Medicine, a Washington, D.C.-based group claiming membership of 3,000 doctors, asked the University of Pittsburgh to stop transplanting baboon livers into humans, calling the experiments "bad medicine and bad science."

It was *deja vu* all over again for Tom Starzl. Once again he was stretching the envelope, seemingly failing but learning at every step, boldly challenging the conventional wisdom. He was once again incurring the wrath of the medical establishment, once again under fire for experimenting with human beings. All the other times, on kidneys, on livers, on new drugs, on just about everything he had attempted, he ultimately made it work and won vindication, but not acclaim, from the medical establishment. If—no, when—the day comes when the shortage of human organs is solved by using animal organs to save lives, Starzl will be vindicated again. This time, though, he may not live to see it.

In a postmortem on the baboon experiments, delivered to a medical meeting later in 1993, Starzl said both men were found in autopsy to be "full-blown chimeras. . . . Baboon DNA was found everywhere, in the heart, lungs, kidney, lymph nodes, skin, and so forth."

Neither patient, Starzl reported, showed any signs of hepatitis B reinfection, or any signs of rejection. And the baboon livers had regenerated well inside the human bodies, tripling and quadrupling in size within three to four weeks.

What went wrong was another mystery, though. In addition to the infections that killed them, both patients had kidney failure and a host of other problems, Starzl reported, including bile ducts that were filled with thickened bile that could block flow.

The findings raised the question, according to a report

on Starzl's talk in *The Journal of the American Medical Association*, of whether a baboon liver may not be metabolically compatible with humans. Starzl said he didn't think that was true, but had decided to back off from any further baboon liver transplant trials "until the issue of metabolic incompatibility is thoroughly resolved." One possible solution, he said, is a drug from a Massachusetts biotechnology firm that might make the human patient less sensitive to the transplanted organ. The drug has already been shown by Duke University researchers to delay hyperacute rejection in some highly sensitive heart-transplant patients.

In addition to xenografting, work is under way on liver cell transplants—where cells from a donor liver are injected into a dying patient's spleen. Research indicates they can begin working and provide improvement to patients awaiting a complete liver transplant. The procedure was first tried in the United States at the Medical College of Virginia Hospitals in Richmond, and was successful, offering what might be an unlimited supply—cells from healthy livers that can be removed and would regenerate in the donor—to help patients in liver failure. (A similar technique is being tested for pancreas transplants, which so far have been largely disappointing. By coating insulin-producing pancreatic cells with "bubbles," researchers believe they can transplant cells without having to suppress a diabetic patient's already depressed immune system.)

And several groups appear close to actually producing an "artificial liver"—a machine that can perform some of the functions of the liver. Such a machine could be used for "liver dialysis," and could form a bridge for dying, waiting patients, much as Leonard Makowka tried to do with a pig liver. In Houston, researchers have been able to grow liver cells on a membrane. By passing blood through the screen, the liver cells do their magic on the blood. Other variations are in research, too, and, according to David Van Thiel, the researcher who

■

went from Pittsburgh to Oklahoma City, an artificial liver may be a reality in a very short number of years.

"I think the artificial liver is begging to be developed and will be developed," said Van Thiel, who has his own project going. He thinks the best use of such a machine will come not with the dying patient in "fulminant" liver failure, but for chronically ill people whose lives could be improved by the machine before the trauma of a transplant. Fulminant patients have so many complications, such as kidney failure and lung trouble, that measuring the success of a liver machine under those circumstances would be a mistake. "Those people need a new-body machine, not a liver machine," Van Thiel said. "I want to build a machine for chronically ill people and bring them into good metabolic balance before transplantation." Such a machine could stretch out the urgency for a transplant and be used as well after surgery to lessen the strain on the new liver.

Van Thiel has been using his machine on small animals—rats and dogs—by inducing liver failure, then hooking them up. Results have been promising, and other groups are progressing as well. "I think it's going to be this year [1993] or next year" for human trials, he said.

Already, though, there had been sporadic uses of such machines with humans. In February 1993, again at Los Angeles' Cedars-Sinai Medical Center, the same place the pig-liver transplant was tried, a thirty-five-year-old woman with end-stage liver disease was hooked up to an artificial liver support system. The patient, not failing enough to have fallen comatose but very sick nevertheless, was eventually transplanted and discharged. That machine, which passes blood plasma through a matrix of pig-liver hepatocytes (liver cells), performs both the liver's detoxification functions as well as some synthetic functions. In kidney dialysis, for comparison, machines only purify blood. This machine, developed by Dr.

Achilles Demetriou and actually first used two years previously at Vanderbilt University, can manufacture the additives that
the liver provides. Each treatment lasts six to eight hours, and
each patient must undergo treatment every eighteen to twenty-
four hours. The experimental treatment is meant only as a
bridge to transplantation, not a full-time liver substitute, the
hospital said. For example, a ten-year-old boy in a serious coma
with pressure building inside his brain was treated with the
machine and stabilized, returning the pressure on the brain to
normal. The boy was then transplanted and later discharged
from Cedars-Sinai.

An artificial liver machine is only part of the battle,
however. It still is a long way from an implantable device that
could take the place of a human transplant. The day of a "bion-
ic" liver may never come, and thus many see the answer in
nature—in genetic engineering and in xenografts.

On the genetic engineering front, Tom Starzl gets a
gleam in his eye that tells you he's dreaming big thoughts
again. "I'm going to see something next month that I can't tell
you about," he said coyly. But clearly, the goal of the most cut-
ting-edge research is not to jury-rig the human body to accommodate an animal organ but to genetically alter the animal
organ so that the recipient thinks the new organ is human.
Such work will undoubtedly lead past baboons to pigs, which
reproduce quickly and with little genetic variation. Pigs are
cheaper, more plentiful, and easier to use since the animal-
rights groups don't attack over pigs as much. They are not furry
and cuddly and, when they are bought off the farm one step
short of bacon, it's hard to argue their lives should have been
saved.

The goal is to somehow come up with a human-like
liver that could be reproduced in pigs. That means genetically
altering a pig liver to take on human characteristics. It's not as
wild as it sounds. A transgenic pig—one carrying transferred

■

genes—that could express human antigens could fool the human body, and already work is under way on such trickery. Baxter Healthcare Corp., the giant hospital supply company, is just one corporation already at work on a transgenic pig. Successfully transplanting a pig liver, though, is probably five to ten years away.

"Pigs are ultimately the answer," Starzl says.

Until the day when the body can be genetically fooled, transplant experts are working to cover the problem up, bury it in the sand of massive immunosuppression. Beyond cyclosporine and FK 506, new concoctions are already in the research pipelines. More power with fewer side effects is the goal. Some drugs are on the way that may work best for certain types of transplants, such as kidneys. And other "designer" immunosuppressives are in the labs, drugs that would enable doctors to suppress the immune system only in regard to the liver, for example, while leaving the rest of the body's natural defenses intact.

By the end of the decade, doctors say, those kinds of magic bullets should be available, once again revolutionizing the rapidly evolving transplant world.

Such work in transplantation may have gigantic benefits for many of medicine's most vexing problems. It turns out that the body's immune system may hold the key to many, if not most, of our most pernicious diseases. AIDS—Acquired Immune Deficiency Syndrome—is a virus that strikes the immune system. And many common afflictions, such as arthritis, multiple sclerosis and diabetes, are connected to the immune system. Some cancers, maybe most, may have an immune-system connection as well, and maybe even an immune-system cure. Spurred by infusions of AIDS-related research dollars and driven by the walking laboratories of transplant patients, who in reality have a chemically induced AIDS-like problem because their immune systems are suppressed, immunology research has been taking off and may ultimately yield heroic and dramatic cures to diseases that have confounded medicine for centuries.

Tom Starzl is one believer. Already he has found that the immunosuppressant drugs—primarily FK 506—he gives to transplant patients have a host of medicinal powers. It turns out that patients with "autoimmune hepatitis"—a disease that attacks and destroys the liver and often leads to a transplant— "have had a high incidence of remission with FK 506 therapy, putting off consideration of transplantation for long periods and perhaps permanently in patients who still have adequate liver mass," Starzl reported to a Paris medical meeting in 1993. Other diseases unrelated to liver transplants also show promise. A large study is under way to determine if FK 506 can help MS patients, for example. The uses of drugs developed for transplantation, and the lessons learned from manipulating the immune system, may well surpass the benefits to the science of transplanting organs.

Reflecting, like a dreamy idealist and an excited researcher, Starzl concluded in one conversation: "There is huge potential for all of this research. Transplantation may end up being only a small footnote to the advances that come from this kind of immune-system medicine. I really believe it may only be a small footnote."

■

CHAPTER 14
THE NEED FOR
ANOTHER MIRACLE

Randy Roady was back in the hospital, but this time it was not Baylor. This time, he was not the patient.

He had begun commuting to Dallas once a week for his checkup in the transplant clinic, driving down Monday, staying in his Twice Blessed House apartment, then giving his blood sample Tuesday morning and going to his appointment with the doctors. After waiting for a possible afternoon phone call with changes in medication or even a return to the hospital, Randy and Cynthy would drive back to Davis Tuesday night to be with their kids.

It had been a long separation, and it had been hard on the children. There were many tears each week, and the parents had found it best to limit the phone calls home to just Wednesdays. Now, things were going back to normal.

No one was really surprised when Heath began vomiting Thursday night, the first full week of January. His cousin, with whom he had been staying, had come down with a stomach bug. Now it was spreading to Randy's kids, and his bigger concern was not catching it himself. As a transplant patient, little things like stomach bugs can be big, big trouble. Even deadly.

By Friday, Heath was better. Cynthy still called the doctor's office and made an appointment for Monday anyway. She was worried about his becoming dehydrated, so she arranged

■

247

for her niece to take Heath in. Monday was a big day for Randy—he had an appointment to get his T-tube pulled, one of the final steps before discharge.

Heath complained of a pain in his side and had fever. His doctor thought it might be appendicitis, so he rushed him to the local emergency room in Ardmore, Oklahoma, to the same hospital where the transplant team had come a few months before on the harvest run that included the stop at the Pink Moose saloon. There, a different problem was discovered. Heath Roady's blood sugar level was a whopping 791. Normal tops out in the one hundreds. No one knew it, there had really been very little warning, certainly nothing that anybody in the family picked up on, but Heath Roady was suddenly diabetic.

Cynthy called the doctor's office from Dallas after Randy's T-tube pull. She got no answer. Strange, where could they be? She began to worry, and then received the news that Heath had been admitted to the Ardmore hospital. She and Randy raced back north, reached Ardmore, found Heath in a room, and chatted with him before he dozed off into a nap. Doctors were rapidly lowering his blood sugar level with insulin injections.

A couple of hours later, Cynthy couldn't wake Heath up. She began screaming to doctors and nurses—he wasn't breathing well either. Heath had slipped into a diabetic coma. Quickly, he was placed on a respirator. And quickly, the Ardmore hospital realized it was in over its head. Heath Roady had to be airlifted out.

The hospital talked to a medical center in Oklahoma City, but they didn't feel equipped to take him. Randy called Baylor, explained the situation, and was told that he would be better off at Children's Medical Center in Dallas, where a pediatric intensive care unit was better suited to the case. Children's tried to have Heath helicoptered out by CareFlight, but the weather was too bad that night. An ambulance raced from Dallas with a Children's medical team aboard. It picked

Heath up and turned around, making the same drive back to Dallas that Randy, and Heath and all the Roadys, had made a few months before with the town escort. This time, there was no excitement, only fear.

The news was worse than anyone imagined. Heath's brain was swelling, which could cause damage. It may have all been the result of the rapid decline in the blood sugar level— Ardmore may have gone too fast on that. Bringing him down slowly might have been safer, doctors said. For now, they put him in a drug-induced coma and paralyzed him with drugs to take any possible strain off the brain and give it time to heal. It would take time, but there was lots of hope this would pass. The long-term concern focused on all the insulin shots Heath faced as a diabetic.

Cynthy Roady was back in an ICU waiting room, worrying herself dizzy. The red-capped Davis Wolves contingent descended on Dallas once again for another Roady. Like father, like son. The grocery store sent peach baskets full of food. Friends and relatives slept in the waiting room, in the apartment at Baylor, in friends' suburban homes.

The vigil was on again.

On Wednesday, Cynthy and Randy met with a doctor. Heath had been there two days, and the coma was much worse. The swelling in his brain had escalated severely. Damage was already evident on the scans and tests. His pupils had become fixed. He was probably going to die.

"We had a lot of hope. Then the doctor said out of the blue, 'If he does live, he'll be a vegetable. And there is a ninety percent chance he will not live,' " Randy said. "We have seventy-two hours to see if he will live. Then the doctor said, 'Don't lose hope.'

"Can you believe it?"

It was every parent's worst nightmare. A dying child, a

helpless feeling. Randy and Cynthy were alone when the dreadful news came. Most of the Davis contingent had begun to return home as hope for Heath had built. Cynthy stayed with Heath in the intensive care unit; Randy wandered to the waiting room.

A friend found him pounding his fists into the wall, screaming, crying.

"Why? Why?

"WHY!"

No one could believe it—it was just too much. After all Randy Roady had been through, after all his family had been through, all the sickness, all the expense, all the separation, all the worry, Randy's transplant experience suddenly looked like a walk in a park. His only son, the son who cried at the door to the intensive care waiting room the night they would not let him see his father, was dying himself—ninety percent chance of that. The ten percent was hardly any better—a brain-damaged vegetable. How much could one man, one woman, one family be expected to endure? The man who was so worried that he'd leave his son with no father suddenly looked as if he was about to become the father without his son. Wasn't this all too much? It was as if the gods, furious at Randy Roady's defiance, were determined to even the score.

"I just want my boy back," was about all Randy Roady could say. "I need a miracle."

Him, of all people. One more miracle.

"This is all a nightmare," Randy said wistfully. "This week, the year. All year seems like a nightmare. I keep thinking I'll wake up, and Heath's eyes will be open."

"If I won the lottery, I wouldn't care. Some things are more important. I'll take health. I just want good health."

Randy was in trouble with the doctors at Baylor, too. He showed up at clinic looking understandably tired and haggled. Where have you been sleeping? he was asked.

"On the floor at the intensive care waiting room."

■

"Not good enough. You have to get a bed there. What have you been eating?"

"Nothing. Candy I guess."

"Not good enough." Bo Husberg read Randy the riot act. There was no sense in putting himself in jeopardy. He had to take care of himself, no matter how difficult the circumstances are, or things would only get worse.

Randy was so depressed worse was hardly fathomable. But he was in a vulnerable, fragile state. Husberg was worried about him.

Instead of waiting by the phone at Twice Blessed House for his lab results call, Randy agreed to call in to the coordinators. He forgot.

Seventy-two hours came and went like a deadline for a death-row inmate. Heath had improved. Doctors had taken him off the medication and tried, unsuccessfully, to wake him up. But he was beginning to breathe on his own, and there was some movement in his eyes. No one knew how much damage there was, though.

"All they say is 'Time will tell,'" Randy said. "It's been a long time now, and they do say, the longer it goes the less chance he has of making it. And the longer it goes, the more damage there will be if he does wake up."

Some terrible questions swirled around the discussion about Heath. If the tests looked bad enough, did the doctors want to put in a feeding tube? Was there any point in life support? Would Randy and Cynthy have to make a decision?

Would they have to make The Decision?

The thought occurred naturally to Randy and Cynthy: Would Heath become an organ donor?

After ten days in the intensive care unit, Heath was breathing on his own and was moved to a regular room. He still had not awakened, still was totally limp, still was a mystery. But he had been given a feeding tube, and long-term-care plans were being made. His brain wave activity, slow and stunted when he came to Children's, was showing much more movement. Instead of a loping curve on the EEG, there were now closer-to-normal up-and-down line squiggles. But a Magnetic Resonance Imaging test of his brain showed some badly damaged areas. There had been strokes, and there had been permanent damage from the swelling. When he did wake up, and doctors now thought there was a good chance he would, Heath would at the least be legally blind and most likely would have memory problems and motor difficulties.

The room was decorated with family photos and pictures of Heath in his football gear with his teammates. There were cards from school chums and a tape player for the cassette recordings from the third and fourth grade classes in Davis. His best friend Josh called every day and got his parents to drive him to Dallas often. The librarian at school sent his favorite book down with a friend. Ironically, Heath's favorite book was *The Broken Arrow Boy*, the story of a boy who goes into a coma after an arrow is accidentally shot through his head. The boy wakes up. Now, the book, propped up on a windowsill, stared back at Heath—one more cruel reminder.

In the room, there was also a sign above his bed: "Hi! I'm Heath. Remember, I can hear and understand everything said in this room. (I love country music.)" Every doctor, nurse and therapist who came to check on Heath would talk to him rhetorically, as if he were awake. "Hi Heath. How you feel today? Pretty lousy, huh?" It was possible, they said, that he could hear and maybe even understand. But, trapped in a shell, he had no way of communicating with the outside world. It was a hard concept to accept, but it offered hope. Cynthy and Randy, eager to grasp any sign of hope, constantly tried to keep him stimulated, moving him around, talking to him, playing his tapes.

After two weeks in a coma, Heath's eyes were open

■

more and more. His body was still totally limp, but he did become more and more agitated, responding to some stimuli. Therapists would come to prop him up for a few minutes or to bend and twist and stretch and exercise his legs. Randy and Cynthy began looking for rehabilitation centers near home in Oklahoma. When he does wake up, they said, he will still need a year or more—who knows how long?—to recover.

A few more days and a little more movement. Did you see that? He moved his legs. Did you hear that? He coughed. "Heath, can you hear me?"

With a tear in her eye and a stiff lip holding back her fear, Cynthy put a present down beside Heath's head: a Dallas Cowboys hat she bought for her football-crazy son to wear during the Super Bowl. Every kid should have a Dallas Cowboys hat for the Super Bowl.

"Wake up, Bubba. Wake up, Bubba," she said over and over again. "I know you're going to wake up."

CHAPTER 15
THE BEGINNING

In early February, the Roadys packed up to leave Dallas again and head north to Oklahoma. Children's Medical Center had all but given up—there was nothing more they could do for Heath. The hospital reasoned Heath was better off in a rehabilitation center or a nursing home than the expensive high-tech specialized hospital. They had done their best to save him, but they had been pessimistic from the start, and now the dire predictions that first week of Heath's crisis seemed so very real: Brain damage, never wake up, vegetable. Being thrown out of Children's seemed a crushing defeat to Randy and Cynthy, who had not given up yet but were finding fewer and fewer signs of hope to cling to. The roller coaster ride of the past year was taking its toll. Randy had prepared for death, then got his transplant, then struggled with recovery and finally turned the corner. Now, an even greater tragedy had eclipsed the family. The Roadys had, for the most part, lost their son. And after believing in medical miracles, they now began to fear that a miracle was not a given.

Insurance was suddenly another battle. Blue Cross/ Blue Shield of Oklahoma, which covered the family because of Cynthy's job as an administrator at a state facility for the mentally retarded, had decided, the same way Children's had, that enough was enough. The insurance administrators told the Roadys they didn't see the need to pay for time in a rehabil-

■

254

itation hospital, when the chances for rehabilitation seemed slim indeed. But Cynthy argued and won a compromise: four weeks in a rehabilitation hospital and no more, unless Heath woke up.

A fighter like his dad, Heath had actually shown additional slight improvement before he left Children's. He regularly responded to stimuli such as pokes and stings, and he could keep his eyes open, though no one knew if he was seeing anything. "Everyone was real impressed," one of his doctors said after the clan departed. But still, there wasn't much there.

Cynthy found a spot for Heath in Oklahoma City, seventy miles north of Davis, at HealthSouth Rehabilitation Hospital. Around the clock, either she or Randy stayed with Heath, talking to him regularly despite the lack of response, bathing him and changing him and exercising his muscles. It was the kind of devotion that perhaps can only be shown between parent and child. There were no questions about what to do, no strings attached. It was simple: As long as Heath was alive, they would never give up.

But life had become an even tougher high-wire act. Randy spent three or four days and nights in Oklahoma City with Heath. Cynthy worked the overnight shift and sometimes double shifts so she could both be home for Hollie and Heather after school and in the evening, and have three or four days off a week to go stay with Heath in the hospital. Around the house, Randy took on the title of "Mom," and Cynthy became "Dad." They played the names for a joke, but it was real to them. She was the breadwinner, he was struggling to be the caretaker. Cooking and cleaning got done somehow, but most semblances of normal family life were gone. The family was still divided, upside down and in turmoil, and the strain was taking a severe toll.

Sitting and worrying around the clock, Randy was gaining weight against the advice of the Baylor doctors. Soon he was as bloated as he had been before the transplant, when his belly had been full of fluid. With Heath's problems, so much of the focus had shifted away from Randy that the transplant was almost an afterthought. Even around Davis, much of the small-town pressure had been lifted off of Randy. "People used to say all the time, 'How ya' doin' Randy?'" he said. "Now it's changed to 'How's Heath?' It took a lot off me, and put it on him. And I'm glad."

Three and a half weeks into Heath's stay at HealthSouth, a therapist brought him a piece of lemon and put it to his lips. To her astonishment, he responded. Soon thereafter, Heath responded to a hug from his mother with a half hug of his own. And that same week, he managed to give Randy a "thumbs up" sign.

The hospital staff was in awe, and the nurses quickly dubbed Heath "M&M"—for Miracle Man. The insurance administrators heard the good news and agreed to extend coverage beyond four weeks, and Heath made rapid progress. His long-term memory slowly came back. His motor skills and his speech progressed in therapy. Soon he could recognize his name, hug his mother, and tell his father, "I love you." Those small steps were all the encouragement anyone needed to race ahead.

Heath had latched onto a purple-and-pink crocheted blanket—his healing blanket. One day, it disappeared. Randy raced to the basement of the hospital to comb through the laundry but could not find it. He returned to Heath's room, panicked at the thought of Heath's heartbreak. After sitting and thinking a bit, Randy went back downstairs and pawed through the dirty linens once again. No luck. He later returned a third time, with still no luck. Then, when he spotted the laundry truck pulling up in front of the hospital, he raced back to the basement a fourth time for one last look. There, on the top of a bin, was the blanket. "You wouldn't believe it," he told Cynthy on the telephone.

"It's in the book," she said.

■

"What?"

"It's in the book—*The Broken Arrow Boy*. The same thing happens to the broken arrow boy."

As much progress as Heath was making, there were still grave concerns, of course. His right side was partially paralyzed. His short-term memory was nonexistent. His communications were labored and difficult. Optic-nerve damage had limited his vision. And he had to be taught all kinds of childhood skills all over again—like using the toilet. Still, the Roadys were euphoric. "He's doing soooo well. We're even going to take him—all the kids—to the circus next month," Cynthy said proudly in June.

"You know," she added. "It looks like we got our second miracle."

Running a farm or a ranch is very much like a giant experiment in ecology and efficiency. Everything must have a purpose; nothing can be wasted. Weeds compete with crops for precious moisture and must be eliminated. The high cost of watering must be balanced against the gain in the crop. The expense of feed for cattle must be balanced against the increase in weight when the cows go to market. Seeds are saved from crops and used next year. Pastures must be carefully exercised for optimal fitness—not to be overgrazed by the cattle and left in poor shape next year yet grazed enough to beef up the cows and stimulate next year's rapid growth. Cows must be bred with just the right lineage to be most productive and taken to market at the optimum time—not allowed to nurse too long on their mothers yet not weaned too quickly. Crops must be harvested at the perfect moment and knowing that point is always a gamble. If you harvest too soon, you may end up with a reduced yield. If you wait too long, you risk disasters such as hail storms or freezes. The whole trick is finding the right balance—the most productive and enjoyable ecology that will keep

■

everything—the land, the animals, and the people—prosperous and healthy.

Such is the ecology of transplantation as well. The whole trick is finding the right balance. Not too much immunosuppression, not too little. Not too much cost, not too little. Do the transplant at just the right time—not too early, and definitely not too late. Find the right mix of patients given the shortage of organs. How old is too old? How sick is too sick? How nice is too nice to turn away?

And after the organ is transplanted, balance the problems with the gains. Hope that by trading one serious condition for another, the patient is trading up.

Don Bryan, farmer and rancher, has learned the lesson well.

Throughout the long recovery—the first growing season since the transplant—Don Bryan struggled to find some kind of balance. He left Baylor in February having emerged from his cocoon of confusion, but all was not particularly well. He had tremendous headaches. He had an infection in one eye that probably had gone untreated too long. But when he finally got antibiotics, they produced, among other problems, diarrhea and threw his liver function numbers out of whack. He was still as thin as a fencepost and lacking in energy. "We are all just having our problems," he said a after a few months back at home.

Still, it was crucial to Don to be back on his farm in rugged west Texas, back to his panoramic view, his house, his dog and, such as it was, back to his own life. More than any new drug or medical trick, the best therapy seemed to be simply gazing out the back wall of windows in the house he and Cathy built, enjoying a soothing, inviting view of the plains that early settlers had likened to the Scottish moors.

"People told me they never thought they'd see him again when we left for Dallas," Cathy Bryan said proudly. "I know he's bad, but you work through it day-by-day. You know, I never thought I'd lose him."

■

Slowly, Don began doing more around the farm, a square-mile spread on top of the edge of the "caprock" south of Lubbock. He began trying to catch up on chores, tend to the fifty cows that graze what was once a cotton farm, and arrange with the government to hold back a chunk of the farm from production in exchange for small payments for the next ten years. In May he bought seed to return the acreage to native grasses, and by Good Friday, he was planting his garden—cantaloupes, squash, tomatoes, watermelons, black-eyed peas, peppers, and pimentos—across a large plot between apple trees, peach trees, and the Bryans' vineyard of Cabernet Sauvignon grapes.

Still he struggled. Trying to weld a repair, Don dropped a piece of red-hot metal down his boot and burned the bottom of his foot, which became infected. More antibiotics were needed, forcing more woes and more adjustments in his other transplant-related drugs. And the headaches continued, keeping him from traveling, working, playing and most of all, returning to his old self. Cathy, frustrated by the team's standard answer that the headaches were probably the result of the steroids and that nothing could be done, made an appointment with a neurologist at Baylor, but held out hope for a simpler cure. In July, Don had a cataract removed from one eye—and the headaches largely disappeared.

After nine months of struggles following the transplant, Don Bryan was finally back to his old weight and, for the first time, feeling more or less as fit as a sixty-three-year-old should. It was the first time in two years, really, that he was feeling like his old grouchy, obstreperous self. And as welcome as the old Don was, the Don that couldn't tolerate college because people were telling him what to read and how to think, there was something different about him, too. The whole experience had changed Don Bryan.

"He's less bitter," Cathy says, and Don agrees.

"I don't go as hard as I used to. I have a new outlook,"

■

he says. "You can't help but think that way when you think I would have been dead."

Having lain in the hospital wondering about his pall-bearers, Don came out of the transplant reviving relations with his children, spending precious time with his grandchildren, and growing to like other relatives he fought with before.

"It's humbled me," Don says. "I'm just so glad to be alive. I really thought I'd never be sitting here talking to you like this."

Cathy is even able to tell tales of the bizarre stunts Don pulled while in his muddled state at Baylor, such as the time he jumped up and down on the scale screaming about his numbers or the time he climbed into the front seat of a car and left the door open. "Don, close the door," Cathy said calmly, only to have him paw at the air between the car and the door.

"Did I do that?" Don asks as the stories are recalled. "Hmmm."

"Sometimes I think they took ten years off him and put them on me," Cathy says.

Actually, Don remembers little from the time he left west Texas for Dallas. The bed-ridden weeks are a blur, the post-surgery days are a fog. Only now, nine months after the transplant, can Don look back and begin to appreciate what his family—mostly Cathy—went through to save his life. "That Aggie can get things done," he said with pride. "I'll never be able to repay all that was done for me."

Each day Cathy reminds Don of a good deed done by the farm implement dealer or the hardware store owner while he was sick or the stack of get-well cards he has never been able to look at, let alone answer. He has also been unable to muster the strength for writing a letter of thanks to the family of his liver donor. "We talk about doing it, but we never do. And we really need to," Cathy says. But there is too much pain, even a year after the fact.

Around the farm, the pressure to bring in a crop each

■

year is gone, easing some of Don's natural tension. Like all farmers, he still frets about rain, and like all west Texas farmers, still watches the clouds for any sign of stirring, any slim chance that a shower might finally come his way. "You never get rain when you need it. If you did, you could get very rich off this land," he says.

The farm used to be Don's father's. For many years Don and Cathy had lived in town, twenty-two miles away in Big Spring, in a big, comfortable home bought with the fruits of Don's petroleum career with Fina. When he retired from that, he had a house framed on the very edge of the caprock and finished it himself—an open, airy, cheerful home, weathered gray on the outside with a tin roof, blond hardwood floors, and a red-brick fireplace inside, all surrounded by a double fence to keep the rattlesnakes and coyotes out. The work was a struggle because it came just as Don's liver disease was becoming worse and worse, leaving him with less and less energy. The house has an Ackerly, Texas, address but Don doesn't like to associate with the tiny down-and-out town, so his checks list his address as "Two Miles West of Vealmoor, TX."

On the farm, Don is a naturalist of sorts. His garden is all organic—no pesticides or fertilizers. As a result, he gets much lower yields from his crops, smaller fruits and vegetables, and more damage from pests. But he prefers the natural state, and he and Cathy use most of the garden for their own consumption anyway. Don also never uses hormones in his cattle. And he prides himself on returning the land to its once natural splendor, with tall, native grasses and rolling hills. The farm is filled with quail and doves and a few endangered bird species, as well as rare Texas horny toads. Even coyotes can get a break on the Bryan ranch. One day, after spotting a large coyote, an animal hated by ranchers and farmers for attacking livestock, pets, and even crops, Don found he couldn't pull the trigger on his shotgun—the coyote was accompanied by three pups.

"You know," Don says, "I can do whatever I want to do

each day and enjoy it. Not many people can say that." If he gets tired working in the barn or building red-brick flower planters for the front of the house, he takes a nap. If he gets thirsty working in the garden, he breaks open a watermelon for refreshment.

For Cathy, life is just as simple and enjoyable. She commutes to her part-time research job in Big Spring at a government soil-conservation laboratory. The former Texas Tech University chemistry major who went off to Miami in 1968 to be a page at Richard Nixon's nominating convention, brings a scientific sense of place and time to the farm, as well as a master's degree from Texas A&M University. For Cathy, like Don, farming is all in making the most of the land, without abusing it, in finding ways to replenish, to improve, while earning a living off the soil. The farm is one big experiment in organics, the chance to respect nature and take advantage of what nature gives.

Most all fifty cows have names given by Cathy, who frets with Don over which ones will go to market. "That heifer is going," Don declares in one instance. "He's not taking her. She's Brownie's daughter," Cathy declares a few minutes later.

"Cows don't take much to maintain. That's why we have the herd now," Don says.

The year of the transplant, Don planted just five acres of cotton, mostly to see if he could handle it. His garden has been for his consumption and for his neighbors and provides food well into the winter after the freezing and canning is done. A single oil well on the property—Bryan One—provides some grocery money, too. Next year, he says, he's going to plant cantaloupes to sell.

Just as they find a natural balance on the farm, so do they find equilibrium in their marriage. He loves to grow things; she loves to cook. He loves to tinker; she loves to study. They both love to read and to sit on the back step and watch for brewing storm clouds, sometimes even doing a little good-

■

luck rain dance to draw the clouds nearer. Most of all, they love to sit on that back step and listen to the silence, to the peace, punctuated only by the call of quail, by a passing dove, the bark of their dog, Sugar, or maybe by the sound of a visiting neighbor's car heard from a half-mile away. They both have a Wallace Stegner sense of place.

"I can't think of anything we need that we don't have here," Cathy says with a utopian passion.

Yet the storm clouds of their lives are never far from thought. "You come to realize that there are things worse than death. I was prepared for whatever would happen. If it hadn't worked out, well, we had our time together," Cathy said one night on the back step, gazing at the stars.

"It's hard to believe where we were one year ago, how far we've come."

What the Bryans have learned is that their lives—Don's second-chance body—now must be balanced just as the farm must be balanced, that nature must be given the same respect for the body as for the land. It is easy to forget that transplantation, like so much of medicine and so much of farming, is simply taking what nature gives you and making the most of it, stepping in to correct things when you have to, when you can, but never forgetting that too much tinkering can lead to trouble.

"If I hadn't had the liver transplant I'd be dead. Think about it. There's no way to say how much it means to you to still be alive."

North of the bustle of Latin Miami, north of the condos and retirement homes of Miami Beach and Boca and Lauderdale, north of the hurricane damage and even ritzy Palm Beach, lies a sleepy Florida coastal community not yet overrun by population—Jupiter. The town has its million-dollar homes and its celebrities (Burt Reynolds, Lee Trevino, and others). It has its

■

beach and its share of the intercoastal waterway, but it also has enough small-town charm left to have country-cooking restaurants and corner grocery stores.

On a corner of a simple, well-kept street sits a simple, well-kept house across the street from an inlet and just over a bridge. The white house has a couple of palms, an orange tree, a strawberry guava bush, a cement roof, delicate landscaping, and a large backyard. Its resident likes to practice his golf swing in the side yard and takes walks every night using a golf club shaft for a walking stick. It seems like it would almost be the perfect retirement spot, laid-back and simple, yet typically Floridian.

For Mel Berg, now sixty-nine years old, it is.

Since leaving Baylor in February, Mel Berg has traveled, enjoyed his grandchildren, seen some old buddies, and knocked twenty strokes off his golf game. He has charged ahead through recovery with the same hard-driving attitude that kept him in relatively good shape before the transplant. Immediately after returning home following seven months in Texas, Mel went to work on his yard, pruning and planting for hours. "The kids were all yelling at me, 'Don't do this! Don't do that!' I just kept saying, 'The liver's not going to fall out.'"

And it has paid off. Berg seems to be a prime example of the dictum that the better shape you are in going in, the easier your recovery will be.

Not that recovery has been all that easy. Mel had excruciating back pain for weeks. Still, he forced himself to walk every night and in five months had pushed himself to two and a half miles per night. He has had chest colds for several weeks, terrifying incidents because of the danger in immunosuppressed transplant recipients of deadly infections. Having grandchildren around the house with runny noses only raised his anxiety. "If my immune system shuts down, you know what can happen," he reminds a visitor. "It was scary coming back here. I wanted to sell this place, or rent it, and buy something in Dallas so I'd be closer to Baylor, real close. It took me about two months to get over the fear of leaving the womb," he said.

The normal routine for transplant recipients for the first year calls for blood work every three weeks and a visit to the doctor every six weeks. The local physician takes responsibility for the patient's care, but many do not yet have broad experience with transplant patients. Lab results are always sent on to Baylor for review, and sometimes the transplant team overrules the local physician. Drs. Husberg and Levy divide the patient pool in half by alphabet but rely heavily on the coordinators to spot suspicious or troublesome numbers. And patients themselves call the coordinators early and often with all kinds of questions, from what to do if a dose of cyclosporine or FK 506 is missed to what to do about a case of sunburn. With the price of the transplant comes a free lifetime service contract.

Six months out, Mel Berg's numbers started zooming up, signaling trouble in his bile ducts and maybe even rejection. What was a frequent routine for doctors became a cause for alarm for Berg, whose liver originally failed because of bile duct problems. But after simply raising his dosage of FK 506, the numbers turned back toward Berg's normal ranges. Mel took it as a sign to never let down your guard.

"Mentally, I'm pretty much set. I'm going to be on guard for the rest of my life with all this blood stuff. But as far as letting me slow down, I'm not going to let anything hold me back," he said. "If I want to move plants, I'll move plants. If I want to go fishing, I'll go fishing, but I hate putting on all that sunblock." (The steroids taken by transplant patients thin the skin and make them more susceptible to sunburn and skin cancer. They also bleed easily from scratches and cuts.)

A bigger concern now are his kidneys. FK 506 and cyclosporine are both hard on the kidneys, and Berg's kidney function numbers have been very high and are climbing. The

■

265

Baylor team, like others, have found themselves considering kidney transplants for liver patients after a few years of the immunosuppressant drug therapy. Many patients are headed for kidney dialysis and long waits for kidney transplants. It is one of the side effects, one of the costs, one of the riddles not yet solved.

Berg tried to find a support group for transplant patients but was surprised when he could not locate one in south Florida. There are a couple of other patients near Fort Lauderdale but not enough for a support group. Liver transplants are still something new to most of the population, especially the elderly population there. Only in the past few years have transplant centers stretched out the age limits for patients. Only recently has there been a liver transplant program in Miami, and it is not yet certified for use by Medicare patients. Besides, for the elderly, chances of success are not nearly as good. Mel Berg is something of a novelty in this neck of the woods.

"I understand I got a second time around here, and I appreciate that fact. I'm not going to do something to jeopardize that. But I'm not going to become an invalid over it."

With that, the natural-born salesman, who was selling shoes door-to-door at age sixteen, has returned to his converted-garage workshop. He's begun fiddling with golf clubs again, even preparing to contact old customers and put out a brochure announcing that he is in business again. Before he fell ill, Berg had an inventory of 1,000 shafts in his modest home and was making 100 sets of golf clubs per year. He would watch each customer play, noting how strong he hit the ball, how fast he swung the club and what imperfections he had in his swing. Then Mel would craft a club to adjust for the way the customer played. The wealthy members of the famous south Florida private clubs loved it, and one of the side benefits was Berg got to play all the great courses for free.

Now, the sixty-nine-year-old transplant recipient is trying to shave his golf game into the 90s, beating sons-in-law, friends, and relatives who play with him. One son lives in the house behind his, another lives walking distance away. A third of the five children is moving back to Jupiter with her husband and two children. His wife, Connie, putters around the house, decorated in peach and green tones with her meticulous paintings, needlework, and quilts. They both keep in touch with several other transplant families they met at Baylor.

It is exactly as retirement should be.

"I never had any expectations. From the time I was told I had to have a transplant, I never worried about it," Mel says. "If you've got a broken arm, get it fixed."

It took five weeks before Arden Lynn, paying her own way, was stable enough to think about leaving the hospital. The infection in her arm turned into phlebitis and puffed to the size of a watermelon but had finally healed—without the ripping-the-whole-damn-thing-out surgery that the vascular specialist was pushing. Her rejection episode had passed, and rejection problems had not returned. Her heart sometimes lapsed into its irregular beat, but the transplant team's cardiologist, Dr. Cara East, had helped control that. Arden contracted the tricky and tough-to-get-rid-of CMV virus common to transplant patients, but a drug called DHPG seemed to be controlling that. Her skin itched, and a slew of specialists just scratched their heads on that one—the best guess was that maybe Arden had some sort of bizarre graft-versus-host disease, where cells from the donor don't mix right and begin attacking her body. All in all, though, Arden was just grateful not to be dead. "I'm ready to get on with my life," she said with a stiff upper lip.

After the five-week-long stay in Baylor, doctors arranged for Arden to go to her daughter's house and to get her intravenous DHPG treatments there. That way, she would have some supervision from Sue, and she would save a lot of money

■

by checking out of the fourteenth floor. That arrangement lasted six weeks before Arden gained enough strength, health, and confidence to return to her own home.

Even then, she was a frequent visitor to the hospital, checking in and out of the fourteenth floor several times. Her white blood cell count fell to 1.0 instead of 5.0 one Sunday, prompting a two-and-a-half-day hospitalization. "I'm really sick of this," she said another day. "My crazy liver tests are off, so I've got to go back in the morning. I want to get to feeling good and going about my business."

Being in the hospital so much kept her abreast of the trials of the transplant team—the bout of food poisoning several patients suffered after a group supper at Twice Blessed house; the pair of open-and-shut transplant attempts on cancer patients, who lost out because the cancer had spread; the death of a man whose wife Arden had befriended. He had gone on the waiting list about the same time as Arden and was in the intensive care unit at the same time as she was. But the man had declined so dramatically before the transplant that he was too sick to recover by the time a liver was found for him; Arden couldn't help but think about what might have been her own fate. It certainly made the continuing nagging problems seem trivial. "I feel so blessed to get the liver when I did and not wait any longer," she said.

On one trip to Baylor, she got to see Dale Distant shortly before his one-year stint was up. To Arden, Distant was the kindest, smartest, most compassionate doctor she had ever encountered—he was also the only one of the surgical fellows, she swore, who could perform a painless liver biopsy. "He was so perfect in everything he did," Arden said. "I told Dr. Distant I was coming to New York for my biopsies if that's where he was going to be. Then I said 'I'm really going to miss you. You have really been a great doctor. But the only thing that bothered me was I could never get you to smile.' He gave me a great big grin and said, You'll be all right.'"

■

On the same trip to the hospital, Arden saw Klintmalm for the first time in several weeks, the first time since she had left Baylor. What he had to say startled her.

"I didn't think you were going to make it. You were one sick patient," Klintmalm told her.

"That kind of talk makes you think," Arden said later.

Trivial or not, the little afflictions kept on after Arden. She suffered from allergies for the first time, maybe the result of a compromised immune system, but they never could figure out what she was allergic too. She had to have a breast biopsy after a lump was found. She fell and couldn't get around for a few days. The itching continued—like a constant case of the chicken pox. And her heart still occasionally started racing, temporarily flipping over into another rhythm, scaring her seriously every time it happened. "I just need to get all of this under control," she kept saying.

Finally, by the end of summer, Arden slowly reached equilibrium. The riddles didn't get answered; she just learned to live with them better. And the rhythms of her world slowly returned. She fiddled around her immaculate house, with the all-news radio station going in the background for company. She began to think about turning Bill's studio into a sewing room. And she found a gorgeous painting of her husband's wrapped in the garage—a view of Rocky Mountain National Park that she had never before seen, but that Bill had painted and wrapped to send off to a National Park Service competition shortly before he died. "Of course I just sat in the garage and bawled," Arden said.

Most important, she resumed her active life with her large book club, a circle of fifty-five life-long friends who have all gone through illnesses, losses, and joys together (and who, unbeknownst to Arden, kept a vigil around the clock outside the intensive care unit while she was there, just to help her family if they needed anything). On a typical day, Arden may talk to twenty of the sisterhood. Several times a week she'll get together with some of them for lunch, or "field trips," or shopping at the mall, or just plain visiting over tea.

"If I never get any better than I am now, I'm better than I was before. I'm not complaining. We're all just so thrilled to be alive that we don't care about all this other stuff. I'm just so grateful to have had the opportunity to have the ultimate gift," she said.

Beyond the life-saving surgery and death-defying recovery, Baylor Hospital had given Arden something else for which she was most grateful: a discount on her bill. Knowing she had cashed in her life savings to pay for the transplant, doctors offered discounts, labs waived some charges, and the hospital offered a cut-rate, blue-plate special. It's not all that uncommon—insurance companies negotiate discounts, and government programs set payment levels at lower rates than doctors charge. It's part of a game, really, like buying a new car. Few pay the full sticker price. For Arden, the result was that her $50,000 worth of insurance was eaten up, of course, but the $100,000 personal check she had written to the hospital to get on the waiting list more than covered the rest. "I kept wondering how long I was going to live on what I had, especially when I had so much extra to contend with," she said. In December, she would qualify for Medicare, and she was now confident in August that she had enough funds to last that long, thanks in large measure to the cajoling and persuading done by Alison Victoria. "They have been so good to me," Arden said of the Baylor staff. Not only did they save her life, they somehow left her with the means to live it as well.

Her insurance company, the one with the meager $50,000 hospitalization policy, had had enough of Arden Lynn, however. They raised the premium she must pay from $350 per month to $683 per month—in an effort, she believes, to force her to cancel the policy. Like a hurricane victim in Florida, Arden has come to believe insurance companies only want customers who never use insurance but only send in money every month. Once you need the insurance, the company doesn't need you.

Closing in on her first year post-transplant, Arden set a special deadline for herself: Get a letter of thanks written to the family of the fifteen-year-old liver donor. She sat down many times with pen and paper in hand. She started the note hundreds—no thousands—of times in her mind. But she could never finish it.

"I don't want to say the wrong thing, but I want them to know what they did for me and for my family," she said. "It's a second opportunity to live on, and the gift from the giver is beyond explanation. How can you thank somebody for your life? I thank God every day. I thank the doctors—I have a litany I go through all the time. I thank the mother of the fifteen-year-old. I even thank the people who made the medicines that make this happen. But every time I try to write, it begins to sound corny. But it's not.

"Now, the harder I try to write the letter the harder it becomes. I want that family to know what it meant to me. I've gone through packets of paper, and it sounds like a thank-you note. That's not good enough. It's not like you can just sit down and say, 'Thank you for the lovely gift.' They should hear from me, and they will."

Toward the end of the year for the four surgical fellows, plans for the following year began to take shape. The job hunt had been a tense one, what with the uncertainty of health care reform on the horizon. But good surgeons were still an important commodity, and these were among the best. Dale Distant agreed to return to the Brooklyn, N.Y., hospital where he had learned kidney transplants to start a new liver program, which he would head. Lars Backman, too, would get his own program—opening Sweden's second liver transplant program. Tom Renard, on the other hand, had decided that his surgical heart lay more in pediatrics then in transplants, and he won a pediatric surgical fellowship at the University of Chicago. And Caren Eisenstein, who had signed on for two years, would replace Backman as Klintmalm's senior fellow. Two other fellows would be selected, returning the team to the normal level of three fellows, since Renard had been a welcome add-on.

Or so everyone thought. Toward the end of her first year, Eisenstein walked into Klintmalm's office and told him she had something to talk about. She said she was unhappy, troubled even. She had an ulcer; she had no life. She had wanted to get into transplants to save lives and even get to know the families she would help. But much of her time was spent with the families of the dying patients, not the living. She hated sitting in the selection committee every Wednesday and making choices over who would live and who would die. It was driving her conscience crazy, she said.

"I couldn't say, 'I'm going to treat you, but I'm not going to treat you.' I just couldn't do it," she said later.

Eisenstein was also increasingly tormented by the donor harvest—stepping into tragedy on a regular basis and carving up humans for their parts. And she was queasy over many of the other issues facing transplant surgeons—such as money and competition for organs.

"GK was very warm and understanding, very compassionate, and I had thought he might be upset," she said. "But he shook his head and said he understood. This was not for everyone. He was troubled by many of the same things. He said he had days when he wondered, too."

Eisenstein had spent six months of her almost year in the laboratory doing research on pigs and handling many of the donor calls at night. It was a hard, isolated life, lacking contact with patients and other doctors. When she returned to rounds and transplant surgery, the team faced some gruesome cases—patients who slowly but inexorably "circled the drain."

Concerned that the profession was training too many transplant surgeons, who naturally wanted to go out and open their own programs and thus stretch the donor supply even thinner, Klintmalm decided to get by for the next year with two brand-new fellows. And he also decided to let Eisenstein quit before the fellows' year ended July 1, so she could have a couple of weeks off.

"I just want my life back. I used to be a fun-loving person. But I changed, and no one knew how unhappy I was the last six months," she said.

"All my life, it seems, I wanted to be a transplant surgeon—since I knew what one was. I went through college and medical school with that in mind. My mentor was a transplant surgeon, and I visited Pittsburgh and UCLA and the Mayo Clinic and came to Dallas because liver transplantation was what I wanted to do."

Then, at a point when she was on the verge of being a highly coveted transplant surgeon, the kind who could command a fat signing bonus from some rich hospital trying to start a new program, Caren Eisenstein decided to quit and do something less stressful. She landed a position teaching trauma surgery at the large county hospital in Fort Worth. Somehow, gunshots and stabbings seemed easier to handle. "The money wouldn't have mattered to me. I just wanted my life back," she said.

The experience at Baylor was one that pushed her surgical skills and challenged her to become a much more involved doctor. She was grateful for all she learned and still believed in the potential for transplants and the results swapping body parts was already producing. She also believed it was not the field for her.

"In transplants, it seemed like the only people you got to know well were the ones who didn't do well. You get to know someone and then they die," she said.

■

"And when they die, they die like dogs, worse than any AIDS patient ever thought. It's horrible to watch. They always die like dogs."

At the end of July, Heath Roady checked out of the hospital and came home to Davis. The Roady's church, two blocks from their house, was decorated for a town-wide party that had been previewed in the local newspaper. Cynthy had baked cakes the night before to feed most of Davis and a sugar-free diabetic cake for Heath. By now, Heath could walk, and though he slurred his words, he could talk with enough enunciation to be widely understood. His vision in one eye had improved to $^{20}\!/_{40}$—good enough to get a driver's license some day with corrective glasses. He tested out at a second-grade level, but the school had arranged for a foster grandparent to accompany him to the fifth grade so he could join his old friends, including Josh, who had stuck by his best friend through day after day of hospital visits.

At the party, Heath wandered around smiling broadly. "Thank you for coming," he boomed over and over again. "Thank you for coming." "Thank you for coming." "Thank you for coming."

Tears streamed down some faces. Few believed they'd ever see the day.

At home, Randy had a surprise waiting for Cynthy— half-a-dozen red roses, a gift from him, and from Heath, for taking such good care of them both. Once again, they had both beat the odds.

"I can't wait to take him back to Children's. I really want to take him back to that hospital and have him walk in and look at all those doctors and say, 'Here's your little vegetable-dead boy,'" Randy said with a touch of anger in his voice, more than offset by pride and gratitude. "Can you imagine— the little vegetable-dead boy walking back in."

If there was anger over the tragedy, and there naturally

■

was, it was reserved for the Ardmore hospital where the coma had set in. Heath would not be going back to Ardmore.

The son they got back was different, though. The old Heath may come back more and more, but it was hard to see. He had been an incredibly considerate child, offering to share his Happy Meal toy at McDonald's with a stranger crying because his had broken. And he used to be a wisecracking practical joker with his father's sense of humor. Now, there was no teasing of his sisters, no tricks or treats, and not as much understanding of his surroundings. Yet Heath had also become much more loving. And his sisters doted over him like never before. "Bubba, can I bring you some popcorn?" "Bubba, what do you want to watch?" The ordeal had brought the children closer, brought them all closer really. Among the many changes, there was no doubt that the Roadys had grown to appreciate having each other much more.

And the father the family got back was different, too. Life was still a struggle for Randy, who had lost some of his playful side along the way. Unable to combat the steroid-induced hunger pangs all transplant patients face, he had gained seventy pounds and was far from taking good care of his second-chance body. Though he had been consumed by Heath's ordeal, he, like many liver recipients, didn't have the stamina to return to work. The National Cooperative Transplantation Study, published in 1991, estimated that fewer than half of all liver recipients were employed—about the same as heart attack and cancer patients. But the study classified eighty percent as "physically active" and noted that part of the difference might be because employers are hesitant to hire transplant recipients.

Randy remained on Social Security disability. When the siren went off for the volunteer fire department, Randy tried to help, bringing cold drinks to his fire-fighting buddies or running gofer errands. He jumped in the chief's car one Saturday and raced out to a four-car pileup on Interstate 35, carrying paramedic Mark Saunders. He helped by ferrying equipment around and directing traffic, but it was painfully obvious to Randy that he couldn't don the heavy, hot fire gear and hold a hose or battle a blaze. "It's not fair to the other guys because they have to pick up more of the load," he said. "I just can't do it anymore."

Still, on this day, Randy did what he could to help a young man pinned inside a small pickup truck. The man, twentysomething and heading north from Texas on a hot summer weekend with a suitcase and clothes in the back and a shiny wedding ring on his finger, got crunched by a trailer-pulling full-size pickup, which flipped over itself. Its occupants escaped with only minor injuries. But the smaller pickup had folded like a squashed aluminum can, and the driver was bleeding profusely from cuts on his head. Mark Saunders climbed into the cab through a shattered back window. With the help of a doctor who had pulled over and stopped, he started an intravenous fluid line while the rescuers waited for a "jaws-of-life" machine to arrive from Sulfur, a nearby town. Randy tried to hurry along gawkers who created a massive tie-up that slowed the arrival of the jaws and an ambulance.

There's a special bond that develops between victims and rescuers at a scene like that. Complete strangers interrupt their lives to take risks and try to save others, all for the sense of community and the hope of making a difference. For Randy, there was an additional bond. He glanced in at the pickup driver, a man struck down even more suddenly than himself, and thought about what they had in common. One minute you're zooming north toward good times. The next you're trapped near death inside a mangled wreck. The fragility of life amazes Randy over and over again. It was a scene he had been at many times as a policeman, a fireman, and an undertaker. Now, though, after all he had been through, there was still a special appreciation for the tragedy.

And Randy couldn't help but wonder whether the man

■

might end up an organ donor that night. It had all the poten-tial—severe head injury in a traffic accident, man rushed to local hospital. If there was swelling inside the brain, there could be serious damage. A liver-transplant recipient naturally won-dered.

"Mark's going to ride in the ambulance. Can you follow him in the car to give him a ride back?" the fire chief asked Randy after the top had been cut off the truck and the man extricated.

"OK, where are they going?"

"They're not going to Sulfur. They're going straight to Ardmore."

Ardmore—home of the Pink Moose saloon, scene of the possible mishandling of Heath Roady's crisis. It would be the first time Randy had been back since Heath was rushed to the same emergency room where his blood sugar was rapidly lowered. After Mark helped wheel the accident victim into a treatment room, blood dripping off the stretcher, Randy ushered his friend out the door and left as quickly as possible. Later, he learned the man had escaped with only a badly broken nose.

For one year, or more, Randy, Don, Mel, and Arden all fought a tumultuous, high-technology battle for life and were left weary and exhilarated at the same time. Everyone lost a friend in combat and yet they all gained a second chance. They were touched by death and yet blessed with life. And they were changed. It had been the struggle of their lives, this war to live. And it had been an enthralling experience to watch how hard other people—strangers—are willing to work to keep people alive. The surgeons, nurses, social workers, and everyone else from Tom Starzl and Goran Klintmalm on down are almost universally left weary by the ordeal of transplantation. They, too, have all lost friends but won more battles than they lost.

For each of the four patients, the ordeal had been far more than they bargained for, and yet knowing all they knew, each would sign up again in a minute. As amazing as the

■

human body is, it turns out the human spirit, the soul, is much stronger. They all emerged from hell tickled to death to be alive, knowing that they won. Winning, hands down, beats the alternative.

If there is a curious footnote, it is that none of the four has been able to sit down and write a letter of thanks to the families of their donors. The words do not come easily; the emotions overwhelm the pen. Transplantation has allowed this unique charity to become standard operating procedure in our society, and yet those touched by it struggle to find ways to show gratitude. How do you thank someone for your life? How do you tell a family still grieving over the tragic loss of a daughter or son, husband or wife, that you are thrilled to be alive, that you are hugging your grandchildren or kissing your wife? How can you possibly explain why you got a second chance and they didn't? How can we deal with such irony, such tragedy? Why do some win, and some lose?

The moral of the story is not that some die but that some live again. Mel Berg gets a reprieve to see his grandchildren and enjoy the retirement he earned. Don Bryan can sit on his back step and bask in the splendor of the silence, enjoying a second chance to grow closer to his children. Arden Lynn can cruise the phones with her book club friends and rebuild her life. Randy Roady watches with a twinkle in his eye as his children grow up and go through school. There is no price that you can put on saving a life or simply adding a few years to one's life. There is no way to adequately thank the professionals and the family that made it happen. It must be enough to know that it does happen, and should happen, and that as the ethical and technical problems are ironed out and health care woes are reformed, it will happen more and more.

Back in Davis, Randy finished a tour for a visiting friend with a drive to the town cemetery he used to take care of, a place where he feels remarkably at ease, a place to which he somehow feels a special bond. He knows almost every headstone and much of the history behind each family. He points out the state trooper who died in the line of duty, and the young girl killed in a traffic accident whose liver was donated for him, and whose funeral Randy worked. He is comfortable in the cemetery in a way many people are not—not just because he dug so many of the graves but also because he has faced death himself, and more than that, because he carries a piece of a dead person inside.

It is a strange, constant reminder.

"I still think I will not live a long life," Randy said, driving around the cemetery. "They say the longest liver transplant is twenty-one years. I'm still in my thirties. I just don't think I'm going to get very old."

GLOSSARY

Anastomosis—The point where two vessels, such as veins, arteries, and ducts, are connected.

Anesthesiology—Science of preventing pain and monitoring the state of the body during surgical procedures.

Ascites—Fluid that accumulates in the abdomen, often because of liver disease.

Bile—The secretion produced by the liver. It is stored in the gall bladder and flows down the bile duct into the intestines. Bile is important for the digestion of fat and contains some waste matter.

Bilirubin—A chemical byproduct from the liver as a result of degradation of cells. Too much in the bloodstream causes yellowing of the skin, or jaundice.

Biopsy—Removal of a small piece of tissue of an organ that can be examined under a microscope.

Bone marrow—Blood-cell-producing tissue inside the bone that manufactures red blood cells and some types of white blood cells.

Brain death—An irreversible condition in which the brain stops functioning while the heart continues to beat.

Cardiology—Science of the heart.

Cirrhosis—A disease where normal liver cells are damaged and replaced by disordered fibrous tissue. Can be caused by alcoholism, blockage of bile ducts, hepatitis, and other unknown viruses and diseases.

Cholangitis—Inflammation of the bile ducts that often leads to liver disease. (In medicine, *-itis* refers to inflammation: Pancreatitis is an inflammation of the pancreas, hepatitis an inflammation of the liver, etc.)

Clotting factors—Substances in the blood manufactured by the liver that help stop bleeding.

■

Cyclosporine—A drug that helps prevent rejection of a transplanted organ by slowing down the body's immune system.

Dialysis—A procedure for removing waste from the body by filtering blood through a machine.

DNA—Deoxyribonucleic acid, the genetic material that contains codes for inherited characteristics. Most genes and chromosomes are made of DNA.

FK 506—An immunosuppressive drug.

Fulminant—Massive, as in fulminant hepatitis.

Gastroenterology—Science of the digestive organs and systems, including the liver.

Hepatitis—A disease that inflames the liver, usually because of a virus infection.

Hepatology—Science of the liver.

Immune system—The complex network of cells and tissues that protect the body from disease by destroying infected and malignant cells, removing debris, and attacking foreign invaders.

Immunology—Science of the immune system.

Immunosuppression—Slowing down the immune system, usually with drugs.

Insulin—A protein hormone produced in the pancreas that is vital to regulating blood-sugar levels. Lack of insulin can lead to diabetes.

Intravenous—IV, the process of giving fluid or medication through a needle inserted into a vein.

Ischemia—Time without blood.

Nephrology—Science of the kidneys.

Neurology—Science of the brain.

OKT-3—A monoclonal antibody or laboratory-made substance that is used to slow and reverse rejection of an organ for a short period of time, usually ten to fourteen days.

Oncology—The science of cancer.

Organ bank—An organization that procures and distributes organs and tissues.

Pathology—The study of cells and tissues in the laboratory.

Pulmonary—Pertaining to the lungs.

Rejection—The destruction of a transplanted organ by the body's immune system.

Respirator—An artificial breathing machine.

Steroids—Medications used to slow the immune system.

Virus—An organism smaller than bacteria that can live as a parasite in cells and cause disease.

Xenograft—A transplant from one species to another, such as a baboon liver to a human.

■

BIBLIOGRAPHY

Transplant History, Background, and Science

Akerman, Jules. "Alexis Carrel: Nobel Prize for Physiology and Medicine." Address by a member of the Medical Nobel Committee, printed in *Transplantation Proceedings*. 1987; XIX: 9–11.

American Medical Association Judicial Council. "Ethical Guidelines for Organ Transplantation." *Journal of the American Medical Association (JAMA)*. 1968; 205: 341.

Billingham, Rupert, and Silvers, Willys. *The Immunobiology of Transplantation*. Englewood Cliffs, N.J.: Prentice-Hall. 1971.

Calne, Roy. *A Gift of Life: Observations of Organ Transplantation*. New York: Basic Books, 1970.

Deaton, John G. *New Parts for Old: The Age of Organ Transplants*. Palisades, N.J.: Franklin Publishing. 1974.

Facklam, Howard and Margery. *Spare Parts for People*. San Diego: Harcourt Brace Jovanovich. 1987.

Goad, Kimberly. "Goran Klintmalm: For Baylor's Transplant Chief, Death Provides Life." *Dallas Morning News*. Pg. 1E. Jan. 5, 1992.

Goldstein, Robert M., et al. "Liver Transplantation, 1990: A Dallas Perspective." *Clinical Transplants 1990*. P. Terasaki, Ed. Los Angeles: UCLA Tissue Typing Laboratory. Pgs. 122–33.

Greene, A.C. *Taking Heart*. New York: Simon & Schuster. 1990.

Gutkind, Lee. *Many Sleepless Nights*. New York: W.W. Norton. 1988.

Hawthorne, Peter. *The Transplanted Heart*. New York: Rand McNally. 1968.

Jurkiewicz, Maurice J. "Nobel Laureate: Joseph E. Murray, Clinical Surgeon, Scientist, Teacher." *Archives of Surgery*. 1990;125.

Kittredge, Mary. "Organ Transplants." *Encyclopedia of Health*. New York: Chelsea House Publishers. 1989.

Klintmalm, Goran B.G. *Transplant Fellows Orientation Handbook*. Baylor University Medical Center. 1991.

Klintmalm, Goran B.G., Husberg, Bo S., and Starzl, Thomas E. "The Organ

Transplanted Patient—Immunological Concepts and Immunosuppression." *The Handbook of Transplantation Management.* Leonard Makowka, Ed. Austin, Texas: R. G. Landes Co. 1991.

Kuss, Rene, and Bourget, Pierre. *An Illustrated History of Organ Transplantation: The Great Adventure of the Century.* Rueil-Malmaison, France: Sandoz Pharmaceuticals. 1992.

Maier, Frank, with Maier, Ginny. *Sweet Reprieve: One Couple's Journey to the Frontiers of Medicine.* New York: Crown Publishers. 1991.

Moore, Francis D. *Transplant.* New York: Simon and Schuster. 1972.

Rapaport, F.T. "Alexis Carrel, Triumph and Tragedy." *Transplantation Proceedings.* 1987; XIX: 3–8.

———. "A Reminiscence: John Marquis Converse—Renaissance Man and Founding Father of Transplantation." *The Chimera.* 1990; 2; Oct. 1990; p. 11–13.

Starzl, Thomas E. *The Puzzle People: Memories of a Transplant Surgeon.* Pittsburgh, Penn.: University of Pittsburgh Press. 1992.

Starzl, Thomas E., Groth, Carl-Gustav, and Makowka, Leonard. *Clio Chirurgica: Liver Transplantation.* Austin, Texas: Silvergirl Inc. 1988.

Starzl, Thomas E., et al. "Cell Migration and Chimerism After Whole Organ Transplantation: The Basis of Graft Acceptance." In press for *Hepatology.* 1993.

Starzl, Thomas E., Shapiro, Ron, and Simmons, Richard L., Eds. *Atlas of Organ Transplantation.* New York: Gower Medical Publishing. 1992.

Stone, Marvin, Klintmalm, Goran, et al. "Chemotherapy and Liver Transplantation for Hepatocellular Carcinoma." *Transplantation.* August 1989.

Thompson, Thomas. *Hearts.* New York: McCall Publishing. 1971.

Warshofsky, Fred. *The Rebuilt Man: The Story of Spare-Parts Surgery.* New York: Thomas Y. Crowell Co. 1965.

Medical Economics and Transplant Finances

Chase, Marilyn. "Medical Quandary: Breast-Cancer Patients Seeking New Therapy Face Tough Obstacles. Many Insurers Bar Coverage for Marrow Transplants as Purely Experimental." *Wall Street Journal.* Pg. 1. Feb. 17, 1993.

Evans, Roger W. *The National Cooperative Transplantation Study.* Seattle: Battelle-Seattle Research Center. June 1991.

———. "Public and Private Insurer Designation of Transplantation Programs." *Transplantation.* 1992; 53: 1041–1046.

———. "Organ Procurement Expenditures and the Role of Financial Incentives." *JAMA.* 1993; 269: 3113–3118.

Evans, Roger W., Manninen, Diane L., and Dong, Frederick. "An Economic Analysis of Liver Transplantation. Costs, Insurance Coverage and

Reimbursement." *Gastroenterology Clinics of North America.* 1993; 22: 451–473.

Evans, Roger W., Manninen, Diane L., and Dong, Frederick B. "An Economic Analysis of Heart-Lung Transplantation. Costs, Insurance Coverage and Reimbursement." *Journal of Thoracic and Cardiovascular Surgery.* 1993;105.

Felsenthal, Edward. "Life-and-Death Medical Cases Drag in Courts." *Wall Street Journal.* Pg. B1. Feb. 17, 1993.

Flynn, Julia. "The Final Option—Radical Surgery." *Business Week.* Pg. 95. Jan. 11, 1993.

Fox, Beverly J., Taylor, Lori L., and Yucel, Mine K. "America's Health Care Problem: An Economic Perspective." Federal Reserve Bank of Dallas *Economic Review.* Pgs. 21–31. 1993.

Levy, Doug. "Organ Transplants 'Lucrative' for Some." *USA Today.* Pg. 1. June 23, 1993.

———. "House Panel Targets Fla. Transplants." *St. Petersburg Times.* Pg. 3B. May 26, 1992.

———. *St. Petersburg Times.* "Serious Questions of LifeLink." Jan. 7, 1993. Pg. 1A.

Smith, Lee. "The Right Cure for Health Care." *Fortune.* Pgs. 88–9. Oct. 19, 1992.

Testerman, Jeff. "Audit Shows Overcharges at Transplant Agency." *St. Petersburg Times.* Pg. 3B. April 14, 1993.

Transplant Issues

Association of Organ Procurement Organizations. "1991 Annual Survey."

Castelnuovo-Tedesco, Pietro, Ed. *Psychiatric Aspects of Organ Transplantation.* New York: Grune and Stratton. 1971.

Dowie, Mark. *"We Have a Donor."* New York: St. Martin's Press. 1988.

Evans, Roger W., and Manninen, D.L. "U.S. Public Opinion Concerning the Procurement and Distribution of Donor Organs." *Transplantation Proceedings.* 1988; XX: 781–785.

Evans, Roger W., Orians, Carlyn E., and Ascher, Nancy L. "The Potential Supply of Organ Donors: An Assessment of the Efficiency of Organ Procurement Efforts in the United States." *JAMA.* 1992; 267: 239–246.

Fox, Renee C., and Swazey, Judith P. *The Courage to Fail: A Social View of Organ Transplantation and Dialysis.* Chicago: University of Chicago Press. 1974.

Khanna, Prerna Mona. "Scarcity of Organs for Transplant Sparks a Move to Legalize Financial Incentives." *Wall Street Journal.* Page B1. Sept. 8, 1992

Kolata, Gina. "Long Waiting Lists for Organs Make Ethical Calls Tough." *New York Times.* Pg. 6. Oct. 18, 1992.

■

Levine, Susan. "Resurrection: How a Weekend of Clockwork Surgery Transformed One Highway Fatality Into Rebirth for Four Critically Ill People." *Dallas Morning News*. Feb. 24, 1991.

McCartney, Scott. "Agonizing Choices: People Most Needing Transplantable Organs Now Often Miss Out." *Wall Street Journal*. Pg. 1. April 1, 1993.

———. "Allocation of Organs Disregards Needs of Patients, May Break Law, GAO Says." *Wall Street Journal*. Pg. B6. April 23, 1993.

———. "Law May Allow Few Transplants for Foreigners." *Wall Street Journal*. Pg. B1. June 30, 1993.

Partnership for Organ Donation. "The American Public's Attitudes Toward Organ Donation and Transplantation." A survey prepared by The Gallup Organization Inc. Feb. 1993.

Recer, Paul. "New Protein Prevents Organ Transplant Rejection in Mice." Associated Press. Aug. 6, 1992.

Sadler, Alfred M. and Blair L., Eds. "Organ Transplantation—Current Medical and Medical-Legal Status: The Problems of an Opportunity." *Proceedings of a Maryland Academy of Sciences Symposium*. U.S. Department of Health, Education and Welfare, Public Health Service, National Institutes of Health. May 24, 1969.

Skolnick, Andrew A. "Transplantation Pioneer Predicts Successful Xenotransplantation Soon." *JAMA*. 1993; 269: 2951–2958.

Thorwald, Jurgen. *The Patients*. New York: Harcourt Brace Jovanovich. 1971.

United Network for Organ Sharing. *UNOS Update*. Vol. 9, Issues 4–6. 1993.

Werth, Barry. "The Drug That Works in Pittsburgh." *New York Times Magazine*. 6, 35:1. Sept. 30, 1990.

INDEX

■